Musings on Perimenopause and Menopause:

Identity, Experience, Transition

Edited by Heather Dillaway
and Laura Wershler

DEMETER

Musings on Perimenopause and Menopause
Identity, Experience, Transition

Edited by Heather Dillaway and Laura Wershler

Copyright © 2021 Demeter Press

Demeter Press
2546 10th Line
Bradford, Ontario
Canada, L3Z 3L3
Tel: 289-383-0134
Email: info@demeterpress.org
Website: www.demeterpress.org

Demeter Press logo based on the sculpture "Demeter" by Maria-Luise Bodirsky www.keramik-atelier.bodirsky.de

Printed and Bound in Canada

Cover photograph: Cleve Wershler
Cover design and typesetting: Michelle Pirovich

Library and Archives Canada Cataloguing in Publication
Title: Musings on perimenopause and menopause: identity, experience, transition / edited by Heather Dillaway and Laura Wershler.
Names: Dillaway, Heather, editor. | Wershler, Laura, 1953- editor.
Description: Includes bibliographical references.
Identifiers: Canadiana 20200375555 | ISBN 9781772582857 (softcover)
Subjects: LCSH: Menopause. | LCSH: Perimenopause. | LCSH: Menopause
—Social aspects. | LCSH: Perimenopause—Social aspects. | LCSH:
Menopause—Psychological aspects. | LCSH: Perimenopause—
Psychological aspects.
Classification: LCC RG186 .M87 2021 | DDC 612.6/65—dc23

Acknowledgements

Heather Dillaway thanks Joani Mortenson for helping to initiate this book and Laura Wershler for making sure we finished it. She also thanks Jason, Aurora, and Teague for putting up with her need to work during family time.

Laura Wershler thanks Heather Dillaway for the invitation to be her co-editor and all the contributing authors for making the editing of this volume a journey of discovery and possibility.

Both editors thank Andrea O'Reilly and Demeter Press for assistance in preparing and publishing this manuscript and the authors for their patience and hard work as we compiled this volume.

Contents

Section Three
BLOOD RELATIONS

10.
Waiting for Seventeen Days
Heather Dillaway

11.
"Dear Magnolia… Nobody Really Understands…
What Can I Do?": Reflections on a Perimenopausal
Blog as Social Support
Gillian Anderson

12.
Finding Bedrock
Marie Maccagno

13.
Menopause Claimed
Laura Wershler

Section Four
UNLEASHED

14.
Harsh Blessings: On Finding Poetry at Fifty
Magali Roy-Féquière

Introduction

A Reading Guide
to *Musings*

Laura Wershler
(with Heather Dillaway)

Where are all the books about menopause? So asks the title of an article by Sarah Manguso that appeared in *The New Yorker* in June 2019. Here, in 2021, is one such book that we believe affirms the subhead below that title: "For women, aging is framed as a series of losses—of fertility, of sexuality, of beauty. But it can be a liberation, too." Aging, specifically women's reproductive aging, is the impetus behind the contributions to this diverse collection about perimenopause and menopause. In these pages, researchers, scholars, poets, artists, and narrative writers explore and expand on the experience and meaning of the menopausal transition. If, as Manguso writes, "we are culturally prepared to perceive women's natural aging as uninteresting at best, pathological at worst—deserving of dismissal or disgust or both," then it is our hope that *Musings on Perimenopause and Menopause: Identity, Experience, Transition* makes clear that women's aging is anything but uninteresting and more than deserving of attention, curiosity, and respect.

What makes this collection unique is the variation in approaches to the subject and the range in emotional tone of the personal experiences conveyed. Between the "hot flash" cartoon at the beginning and a woman's musings about "all new panties" at the end, readers will find a stunning array of quantitative, qualitative, analytical, and introspective detail. What might strike one reader as positive, may be perceived by another as negative. What makes one reader laugh, may make another cringe. This variability in how women think about the menopausal transition when they actually go through the experience—how it becomes richer and more complicated, messy, or eye-opening in both positive and negative ways—is the defining characteristic of *Musings*.

Although the established clinical definitions of perimenopause and menopause permeate the pieces in this volume, they do not dictate the course of these narratives, scholarly or otherwise. Most women are now familiar with the distinction between the two. Perimenopause refers to the period of time leading up to menopause, when signs or symptoms— such as irregular bleeding, hot flashes/flushes, insomnia, and others— may begin, often lasting several years before the end of menstruation. Menopause is reached once twelve consecutive months have passed without menstrual flow. The median age at natural menopause for White women in industrialized nations is between fifty and fifty-two.[1] Post-menopause is used by many[2] to refer to the phase following the point at which menopause is reached, whereas others[3] suggest the words "postmenopausal" and "postmenopause" are redundant—that to reach menopause is also the start of living in menopause.

Feminist researchers and writers have long proposed that how women recognize, define, and cope with their own experience of perimenopause, menopause, and postmenopause is just as important, if not more so, than how their experiences intersect with these tidy clinical definitions. Individual women recognize reproductive aging as an important life-stage transition, not just as a retrospective moment in time or as a clinical diagnosis. Furthermore, although biomedical and feminist researchers agree that reproductive aging is a time of transition and border crossing, they offer differing perspectives about whether menopause signals deficiency and burden, or growth and freedom, or both. Contributors to this volume address both and also something more entirely. Research, analysis, inquiry, narrative, poetry, and art intermingle to create a multitextured montage that challenges stereotypes, probes relationships, and reframes traditional touchstones of the peri- to postmenopausal experience.

At first glance, the collection defied categorization. But as we worked through the editing process, unifying ideas emerged that crossed format boundaries and suggested how best to present this assorted anthology. The volume is divided into four parts, titled by theme.

One: Meno-Typical

In this section, the contributors approach, in both conventional and nonconventional ways, the typical talking points and issues of concern around the menopausal transition. By "typical," we refer to the biomedical discourse that has become a "master narrative" (Lyons and Griffin) of sorts, constructed by the information we receive from family, friends, healthcare providers, and lay culture. No one can deny that menopause and reproductive aging have been medicalized and pathologized such that most women have internalized ideas about negative symptoms and absorbed information about safe and/or effective treatments. As we discuss again in the conclusion of this volume, the focus on bodily symptoms and markers of this change as well as the reliance on doctors and researchers as experts (rather than women themselves) can potentially lead to initial negativity and uncertainty. But as the pieces in this section attest, women also come up with their own ways of negotiating bodily symptoms and reinterpreting what these experiences mean for them.

Take one of menopause's most prevalent and enduring tropes. In the opening piece, "The Anatomy of a Hot Flash," Beth Osnes uses cartoon images and expository captions to interpret a personal yet almost universal experience, one she perceives to be both disruptive and liberating. The duality of her perception is a recurring theme in most of the chapters of this book.

In investigating both the biomedical and psychological factors related to the menopausal transition, Mary Jane Lupton provides a sort of postscript to the seminal work she co-authored over forty years ago. Her intention for the chapter in this book is to "review, rethink, and update what we wrote" about menopause in *The Curse: A Cultural History of Menstruation*. Riffing off popular culture throughout the piece, she uses "gone girl" imagery and metaphor to both inform and satirize the cultural history of menopause: "Among the contemporary middle class, the postmenopausal woman is the gone girl veiled in the cloak of invisibility and past her prime."

The master narrative about menopause can affect not only how we experience it but also how we anticipate this life-stage transition. In "Myths and Misconceptions," Jane Ussher, Alexandra Hawkey, and Janette Perz present research into how migrant and refugee women construct and experience menopause. Although most women were premenopausal at the time of their interviews, they foresaw as negative the most expected bodily changes associated with the menopausal transition. Yet across cultural groups, some women challenged negative constructions of menopause. Access to accurate information following migration was one factor that led to more positive outlooks. As one woman said: "I used to hear about menopause. When the menstruation stops, the woman feels that her age is now come to an end, and she suffered depression, but here in Canada, they don't think [this] about menopause. After menopause, life starts." Others described menopause as a "natural process" or just "another stage" of life. This, too, can be considered a typical perspective on menopause.

Mindy Fried's personal essay, "The SWAN Study: Gender, Race, Identity, and Menopause," broadens the frame as she intertwines her experience as a participant in the longitudinal Study of Women's Health Across the Nation (SWAN) with data on race, culture, and identity drawn from the study's findings. A sociologist and experienced researcher herself, she is struck by how SWAN gave her a regular opportunity to reflect on the process of growing older. It also alerted her to information about her own health, including issues associated with the menopausal transition. To these personal benefits, Fried adds the potential for the study's data, collected from a diverse population of participants, to improve the lives of aging women.

It is a poet's voice that ends this section. In "Slouching towards Menopause," Joanne Gilbert personifies the unwelcome visitor that shows up just when she thinks the endpoint is near:

> I wasn't glad to see you
> after almost a year of
> living without you.
> Your return, unbidden, unwanted
> unhinged me

With sustained metaphor, Gilbert poignantly captures the uncertainty many women "typically" experience during perimenopause.

Meno-Typical establishes the master narrative as a foundational reference point. From here, the collection branches out to extend the reach of menopause discourse.

Two: Out of Step

Out of Step shifts direction with stories that fall outside normative experience, where the transition to menopause does not happen at the age or in the way it is expected to happen. These pieces challenge our top-of-mind ideas about menopause, about aging women. We learn about a medical condition, primary ovarian insufficiency (POI), from both clinical and personal perspectives. In "Before Your Time: When Menopause Comes Too Soon," the voices of young women pierce the narrative that perimenopause and menopause are experiences reserved for women in midlife. Co-authored by medical sociologist Evelina Sterling, an adolescent health physician, and two patient advocates, this chapter weaves together facts, figures, and health issues with the words of young women experiencing POI. One woman, age thirty-seven, said the following about her experience with POI:

> My diagnosis was unexpected and unwelcome. Nevertheless, my POI had a strange, uplifting effect on my life. I now recognize the importance of life and what a gift it truly is.... Don't get me wrong, like probably all women with POI, every day that goes by, I continue to wish that my diagnosis could be reversed. Yes, I still long and wish for my fertility back. Yes, I worry about my hormone levels, my bone loss, my early aging, and all the other things that come along with POI. But now, I see every day as a learning day.

Yolanda Kauffman, a social worker and contemplative photographer, intermingles images with words to offer an individual perspective on too-early menopause. In the preface to her chapter titled "Shadow Story," she notes how her creative practice helped transform "a devastating and painful thirteen-year event into a mystical and powerful experience" of growth and learning.

Award-winning poet Donna J. Gelagotis Lee begins her transition story, at age forty-one, with a medical pronouncement—the kind that probably has given many women false ideas about how and when most of us reach menopause. Not suddenly, at some predetermined age in the early fifties, but through a series of bodily and other changes over a progression of years:

Forty-one
Too young for menopause, the doctor says
as I look at a picture of his wife, almost
my age, and wonder what he'll be telling her
if she wakes up in a sweat one night

In stanzas titled by age, year by year up to fifty, "Just before Menopause" takes the reader through a perimenopausal tour of curiosity and uncertainty. Lee's poetic exploration questions and discovers, ponders and reflects, in ways that will resonate with many.

What about an early menopause that isn't really menopause? Georgiann Davis, a woman with complete androgen insensitivity syndrome, recounts her "psuedo-menopause" experience in a compelling story that begins as follows: "Menopause often marks a transition in a woman's life, as it did for me ... only I was a teenager when doctors surgically shaped my body leaving me in what they labelled 'postsurgical menopause.' I was born intersex, but like other intersex people, I wasn't told the truth when I was diagnosed." In "Patches Not Pads: An Intersex Experience with Postsurgical (Pseudo) Menopause," sociologists Davis and Koyel Khan draw on Georgiann's intersex experience to make the case for holding doctors accountable for their constructions "of both intersex and menopause status." The authors touch briefly on voices missing from this volume by asking questions about how the lived experiences of trans men and women might add to the discussion of socially constructed menopause.

The pieces in this section see beyond the master narrative of menopause to a broader narrative framework that includes these seemingly out-of-step experiences. If we reconceptualize meno-typical to include the atypical, we can grasp the range of identity and experience possible during the menopausal transition.

Three: Blood Relations

When thinking about our own reproductive experiences, we use our connections with others as both a guide and sounding board to help us interpret and negotiate these experiences. Relationships matter, and connections with others shape how we see ourselves. The pieces in Blood Relations explore how relationships of various kinds—mother and daughter, woman and partner, women helping women—influence perception, decision making, identity, and sense of community throughout the transition to menopause.

Our contributions to this volume, which open and close this section, explore the mother-daughter connection from different directions. In "Waiting for Seventeen Days," Heather Dillaway shows us the intimate bodily knowledge that may exist between mothers and daughters. When she and her daughter download an app to chart their menstrual cycles together, an unexpected perimenopausal event catches her off guard: "The most jarring part of the lateness was that I had been looking forward to using the period-tracking app with my daughter. I was almost ashamed to tell her I had nothing to track. Being seventeen days late that month meant being unlike her, when I thought we now were moving in parallel." Finding the coincidence of her daughter's menarche and her perimenopausal event "clarifying," Dillaway discovers another point of commonality: adjusting to their respective evolving life stages together.

In "Menopause Claimed," Laura Wershler explores how a workshop experience revealed previously hidden significance in the reproductive connections between herself and her mother. She describes how her mother's loving presence seeped into each memory that surfaced in a guided visualization through the "blood rites," from menarche to menopause, sparking this insight:

> What stuck in my mind was the recent loss of my mother.... I was still recovering from the physical and emotional exhaustion of being her primary family care provider, of watching my beloved mother struggle with advancing frailty. I realized at that moment that only when she was gone, when I was sixty years old, did I feel as if I had finally reached menopause.

Wershler comes to appreciate the interconnectedness between all women (not just between blood relatives), whatever our experiences with the blood rites might be.

Evolving relationships with her partner and adult children form the backdrop to Marie Maccagno's quest to transform her relationship with herself. In "Finding Bedrock" she travels both inwards and outwards, seeking a foundation on which she can ground her life. She starts from a place of deep vulnerability: "For many weeks, I felt as if I was living behind plexiglass, a see-through barrier keeping me apart from the life going on around me. My nerve-endings felt numb, my thought processes like thick mud sliding slowly down a shallow slope. Questions about my future circled endlessly in my brain." Disoriented by an unexpected diagnosis and a major relocation, Maccagno leans into her rich connection with nature. Walking—through forests and mountains, over roads and trails, on the Camino de Santiago—and writing become pathways to a new way of being with her family and herself.

Beyond familial relationships, friends and peers also serve as a benchmark. The identities and experiences of others can help us interpret our own, as we see in "Dear Magnolia," Gillian Anderson's in-depth analysis of *The Perimenopause Blog*:

> A central and organizing narrative evident in "Dear Magnolia" is perimenopausal women's desire to connect with other women at this stage in their lives. They want someone to talk to, to listen, to relate to, and confide in. Someone they can share their feelings and experiences with. Women want support and are online actively creating or searching for a sense of community.

Anderson recognizes the online support community developed by Magnolia Miller "as part of the larger historical record of how women use their relationship and community-building skills to support one another during transitional times."

The personal and collective narratives in Blood Relations illustrate how our social-emotional relationships influence, contribute to, and help us make sense of our transitional experiences.

Four: Unleashed

The last section explores how women "unleash" themselves from expectations, societal norms, and assumptions about the aging reproductive body. These pieces are about seizing the freedom to be, to create, to push boundaries. Through both ordinary means, like needlework, and transgressive actions, like an illicit affair, we see how women can reimagine their lives, challenge what is expected of them, and take risks that may or may not pay off.

In "Harsh Blessings: On Finding Poetry at Fifty," Magali Roy-Féquière explores how "the fresh perceptions" that menopause thrust upon her unleashed her poetic soul. This gender and women's studies professor writes: "Before menopause, I had no idea I could create with words." Distilling impressions and experiences from a period of dis-orientation she calls both exciting and sad, Roy-Féquière expresses her newly accessed creativity in a series of poems forged with vivid imagery and visceral language.

Philosopher Sylvie Teillay-Gambaudo digs into issues of gender, phallogocentrism, and dominant medical discourse in "Uninhabitable Lives," making a case for why we need female-centred narratives on "what menopause actually feels like." Her in-depth analysis of two films examines what are considered to be transgressive behaviours and the consequences unleashed for the characters involved:

> While seeking cinematographic narratives of menopause ex-perience, I was struck by how frequently aging experience was depicted alongside, or enmeshed with, other experiences that could be categorized as uninhabitable.... I will discuss how the aging narratives in *Notes on a Scandal* and *Carol* are presented in a dynamic of mutual support with other narratives: criminality and aging on the one hand and homosexuality and aging on the other.

Women's experience, she concludes, has the transformational power to "render visible those experiences that social conventions conceal."

Victoria Team's chapter, "Perimenopause: The Body, Mind, and Spirit in Transition," conceals nothing, providing the reader with a first-person, real-time account of one woman's topsy-turvy journey through the stages of perimenopause. Team invokes the diversity of her life experience to tell a story full of wonder, dismay, confusion, family, and spirituality. She unleashes vulnerability to share embarrassing incidents: "Once at a social gathering in a café, I had a hot flush and dizzy spell, felt a massive uterine wave, and noticed a stream of blood running through the mesh chair to the floor." She unleashes honesty to disclose actions at odds with her strongly held Christian beliefs: "I appreciated and sought compliments. This desire was so strong that I actively tried to attract people to whom I was not attracted myself." She unleashes her desire, at age forty-eight, to prove she has not lost her reproductive ability: "Something powerful compelled me to try to get pregnant again." As a doctor, she unleashes her medical training to seek answers and solutions to confusing physical symptoms but to no avail: "I am a health professional, yet I misinterpreted perimenopausal symptoms that I experienced, attributing them to an unknown serious illness." By conveying the complexity of her own perimenopausal transition, Team assures those who may have similar experiences that they are not alone.

One of the most well-known feminist works of art is the subject of Anne Barrett's essay "From the Crowning to the Crone: Extrapolating Judy Chicago's *Birth Project* to Older Women." Her essay "examines the broader implications of the *Birth Project* for revisioning women's lives beyond their youth and outside of their reproductive lifecycles." Barrett explains that Chicago herself hinted at a more expansive understanding in her writings about the project, pushing beyond the conceptual confines of women's reproductive capacity. In addition, excerpts from the journals of participating needleworkers suggest the act of creating images for the project had powerful lasting effects on their own lives. As one wrote: "It seems that being part of the *Birth Project* has unleashed our energies in many ways. Who would have dreamed that a 'sewing circle' would become so revolutionary!" Barrett's fascinating analysis of the parallels between the archetypes of the mother and the crone extends the revolution from birthing bodies to aging bodies.

To conclude this section, and the collection, we chose Cayo Gamber's charming piece "All New Panties." With humour and exuberance, she sets us down on the positive side of menopause:

> I looked forward to menopause because I decided that once menses was safely behind me, I would buy all new underwear and not have to worry about any more stains. Once menopause was assured, I went online and discovered, to my delight, that the choices for women had changed over the years. I spent two hours shopping for underwear. In the end, I still bought 100 per cent cotton briefs, but I was able to find underwear that had fun designs—Mondrian squares, Kandinsky colourful compositions, prosaic plaids, pastels and fluorescents, even a Hello Kitty, which I loved for the implied double entendre.

Unleashed in the most practical of ways.

Guided by these four themes—meno-typical, out of step, blood relations, and unleashed—we have compiled the collection to present what we think is an intriguing diversity within each section. Several pieces touch on more than one theme, testament to the complexity of the experiences they recount and the analysis they provide. You might choose to read this book one theme at a time or skip around from here to there according to your interests or field of study. Whatever path you follow through *Musings on Perimenopause and Menopause: Identity, Experience, Transition*, expect to glean how profoundly one's sense of a reproductive life, identity, or intact body, or one's relationships with others, can influence how women process their respective menopausal experiences.

As editors, we thank our contributors for their patience and gracious support throughout the finalizing of this volume. Their scholarly, thoughtful, honest, and compelling work helps us better understand how women think about and experience the menopausal transition in contemporary times.

Endnotes

1. For an in-depth discussion on age at menopause see "The Timing of the Age at Which Natural Menopause Occurs," by Ellen B. Gold.

2. As of August 2020, WebMD refers to the time of a woman's life following menopause as postmenopause.

3. The Centre for Menstrual Cycle and Ovulation Research (CEMCOR), housed at the University of British Columbia, Canada, considers postmenopause to be "an old-fashioned, inaccurate and repetitive way of describing menopause."

Works Cited

Gold, B. Ellen. "The Timing of the Age at Which Natural Menopause Occurs." *Obstetrics and Gynecology Clinics of North America*, vol. 38, no. 3, 2011, pp. 425-40.

"Glossary." CEMCOR, 2021, www.cemcor.ca/resources/glossary# letter_p. Accessed 23 Feb. 2021.

Lyons, A. C., and C. Griffin. "Managing Menopause: A Qualitative Analysis of Self-Help Literature for Women at Midlife." *Social Science & Medicine*, 56, 2003, pp. 1629-42.

Manguso, Sarah. "Where Are All the Books about Menopause." *The New Yorker*, 24 June 2019, www.newyorker.com/magazine/ 2019/06 /24/where-are-all-the-books-about-menopause. Accessed 23 Feb. 2021.

"Postmenopause." *WebMD*, 2021, www.webmd.com/menopause/ guide/menopause-living-managing. Accessed 23 Feb. 2021.3

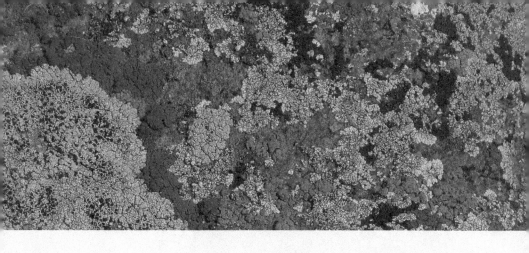

SECTION ONE

MENO-TYPICAL

Wherein women react, in both conventional and unconventional ways, to the "typical" talking points and issues of concern about the menopausal transition.

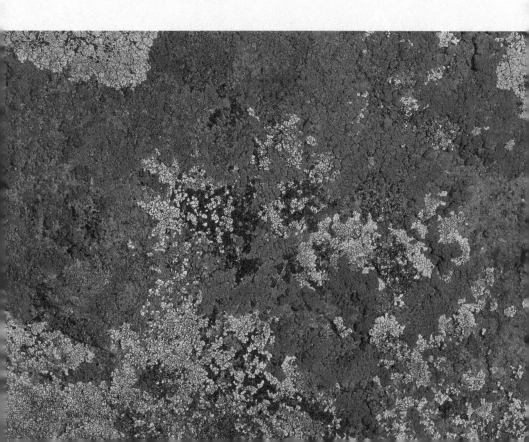

Chapter 1

The Anatomy of a Hot Flash

Beth Osnes

Anatomy is the study of the structure of something, its internal workings, the separate parts revealed through dissection:

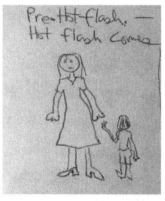
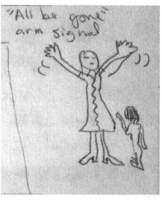
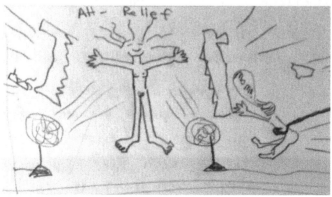

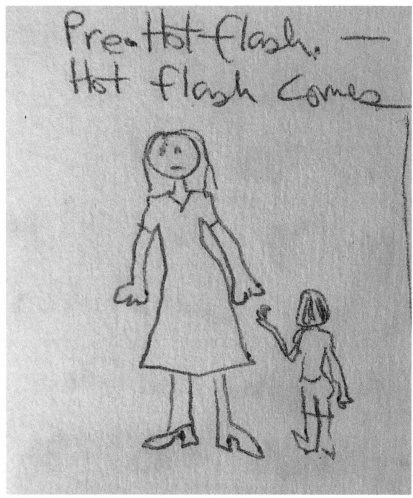

1. Pre-Hot Flash: The specimen is standing content with her child. Maternal allegiances are intact as the maternal unit reaches for the outstretched hand of the dependent child. There is a calm demeanour hovering over their union. The status quo is intact. The societally expected mother behaviour of providing unpaid care for the dependent child is happily provided by the mother. However, as the caption notes, a hot flash in the perimenopausal mother unit threatens to disrupt all of this.

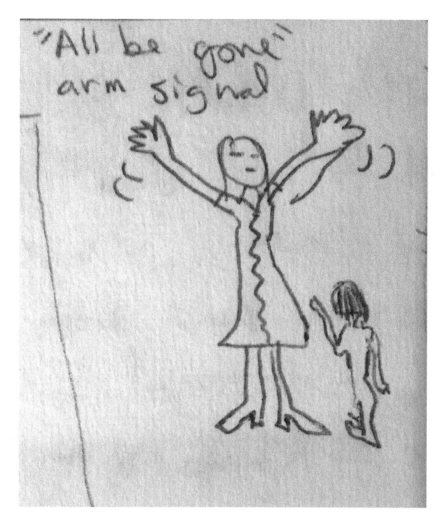

2. All Be Gone: Here, we see the maternal subject raising her arms to make a rather majestic arm gesture, showing her desire for all outwards stimuli, including the dependent child, to be gone. As indicated by the still outstretched hand of the child, the unfulfilled grasping of their hands is left in limbo, with hope on the child's part still highlighted by the muscular effort necessary for the persisting extension of the arm. What we cannot see is the mother's temperature rising and the resulting explosion of claustrophobia through her entire being; she feels not fear so much as irritation with being confined in this role, this moment in time, and even in this garment. Note the beginnings of a disfiguration of the fibres in a zig-zag preparation for release.

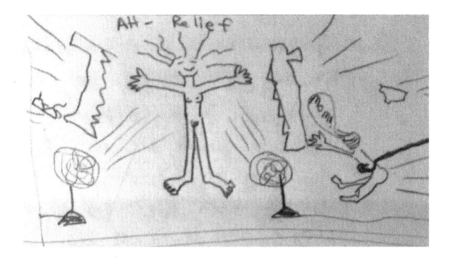

3. Ah, Relief: Here, we see the fulfillment of the inner longings of the maternal subject during a hot flash—her garments are flung wide, her child is quickly removed, and her hair is blown into a lion's mane. Circulated air blasts her with its cooling effects across the geography of her naked body. Pleasure from the release of her confinement overflows from her facial expression. Outwardly, there is something chaotic about this entire scene; it is disruptive yet emancipatory. Inwardly, the desires of the maternal subject are privileged and fulfilled.

Chapter 2

Gone Girl: The Menopause in Popular Culture

Mary Jane Lupton

More than forty years ago, Janice Delaney, Emily Toth, and I unearthed a myriad of works of literature and popular culture, some obvious and many disguised, about menstrual blood and its significant absences. What resulted was *The Curse: A Cultural History of Menstruation* (1976), which is still available in an updated second edition published in 1988 by the University of Illinois Press. All references to *The Curse* in this chapter are to the Illinois edition.

The Curse, which outlines many misconceptions about menstruation that emerged in the medical community over the past two centuries, examines and interprets references to the menstrual cycle in poetry, fiction, and popular culture. We observe that although menstruation has been signified by the flow of blood and by an assortment of symbols—such as flowers, rivers, the colour red, and the moon—and that the first appearance of menstrual blood has been frequently celebrated in tribal or private ritual, the menopause, the final phase of the menstrual cycle, has been given far less attention. Commonly depicted as the crone, the witch, or the hag, the postmenopausal woman was once persecuted for having survived her ovaries (43-44). She was the archetypal "gone girl."

Although male writers, from Homer to Chaucer to Shakespeare, have had the authority to chronicle the condition of the aging woman, they had no technical term for her; the word "menopause" did not come into the English language until the end of the nineteenth century (225). The most notorious of the deviants was Gertrude, the over-sexed mother of

Shakespeare's Prince Hamlet, whose middle-aged remarriage caused the collapse of the state of Denmark (227).

Among women writers, British poet Elizabeth Barrett Browning was perhaps the first to describe the feelings of loss and sterility accompanying the transition towards menopause, what is now recognized as peri-menopause. In *Sonnets from the Portuguese*, Browning, then thirty-nine, expresses her fears that she would be too old for a fruitful marriage. In Sonnet 4, she compares her body to a dilapidated house; the windows are broken, and bats are living in the roof. Images of dust, dryness, aging, inferiority, and sterility occur frequently in Elizabeth Barrett's sonnets and in her letters to Robert Browning, revealing her fears of sexual inadequacy as she approached her fortieth year (Lupton, *Elizabeth Barrett Browning* 32-37; *The Curse* 225).

Like Elizabeth Barrett Browning, American poet Anne Sexton links her physical deterioration to her fortieth year, describing the menopausal transition as "the November of the Body." Her two days of menstrual bleeding indicate her womb's failure to bear a son. Images of a bleeding corsage and blighted buds coincide with her seasons of harvest and death (*The Curse* 192).

The poet Lucille Clifton has written extensively about menstruation and the menopause. In "poem to my uterus," she anticipates the artificial menopause that will follow her hysterectomy, calling the uterus a "sock": "You have been patient/as a sock/while I have slippered into you/my dead and living children/now/they want to cut you out" (*Collected Poems*, 380). In a companion poem, she compares her uterine "sock" to a messy brown bag from which her six children had emerged. Clifton's final farewell to her uterus, "to my last period," begins: "Well girl, goodbye/after thirty-eight years" (*Collected Poems* 381; see also Lupton, *Lucille Clifton* 103-07).

In writing, in ritual, and in popular culture, the menopause has generally been overlooked or rarely underscored as a significant phase in a woman's reproductive life. This current chapter intends to review, rethink, and update what we wrote in *The Curse* about the menopausal transition, with an endpoint generally thought to occur in the early fifties, but whose length and indeterminate quality show that many women, frustrated by the inconclusive nature of this final reproductive cycle, are unable to ascertain when it begins and when it might ever finally end (Dillaway and Burton 168).

The scientific community has viewed the menopause as both a natural phase in a woman's life and a sign of disease and contamination. Doctors in the nineteenth century often treated the "change of life" by attaching leeches to a patient's neck or by performing venesection (that is, bleeding, usually from the arm) to remedy the body's failure to discharge excess blood (Delaney, Lupton, and Toth 216). Many experts, then and now, have connected the menopausal transition to hot flashes, flabby breasts, and a loss of sexual desire. They have also related the hormonal shifts of progesterone and estrogen levels during perimenopause to cancer. But decades of research on whether these hormones (our own or synthetic forms found in hormone therapies) increase or decrease the risk of cancer or other diseases have not led to a definitive consensus. For example, Google "Does estrogen cause breast cancer." The diversity of conclusions drawn is confusing.

The primary twenty-first-century remedy for the symptoms of the menopausal transition is hormone replacement therapy (HRT), more currently referred to as hormone therapy (HT). This treatment that has appeared in various forms—from conjugated estrogen tablets, to wild yam complex, and other menopausal herbs, such as Drenamin, to a product called Estring, a soft, flexible, cream-free ring which, when inserted into the vagina, releases a local, low dose of estrogen.

Obviously, women are still confused, as they were when we wrote the first edition of *The Curse*, about the risks and the benefits of hormone therapy. Even the manufacturers who have promoted the bestselling drug Premarin warn about its potential side effects, which include "abdominal pain, asthenia, pain, back pain, headache, flatulence, nausea, depression, insomnia, breast pain, endometrial hyperplasia, leucorrhea, vaginal hemorrhage, and vaginitis" ("Premarin").

In her evaluation of hormone therapy, Dr. Christiane Northrup takes a balanced approach: "After decades of trying to convince all women that menopause was a deficiency state that could be 'cured' by hormone therapy, we finally realized the truth. There is no magic bullet, one-size-fits-all hormone prescription or drug regimen of any kind that is right and healthy for all women to take indefinitely" (156). In her opinion, bioidentical hormones—which are hormones made in a lab from "hormone precursors found in soybeans or yams" (153)—are far preferable to synthetic estrogens such as Premarin, which is made from the urine of mares. Almost every study I have consulted is suspicious of such drugs as Premarin or Provera for being promoted as cure-alls for the symptoms surrounding the perimenopause.

Many women who have participated in menopausal studies have revealed that they experienced none of these symptoms and that the irregular and then final absence of menstrual blood was a blessing. *Curse* co-author Emily Toth emailed me that although she did experience hot flashes, they occurred only at night: "It was the only time in my life when I wasn't freezing." Gone was the fear of getting pregnant. Gone was the need for menstrual products. Gone was the girl we all used to be.

Gone—but perchance to return? A team of researchers in Greece has claimed to be able to "rejuvenate" women's ovaries and has "reversed menstrual cessation in multiple women," including one forty-year-old whose period had stopped five years earlier (Fenton). The Greek scientists have hypothesized that fertilized eggs could be implanted in the uterus, but they have yet to perform the necessary tests Although the language of hormone therapy has shifted, from HRT to HT, there still remains the hint of the estrogen-generated fountain of youth promised by Robert A. Wilson in 1966: A woman could be feminine forever.

Articles and books about the perimenopause explore its most common symptoms: hot flashes, bloating, cramps, dryness of the vagina, uncertainty about the use of estrogen, confusion, dementia, or down-right madness. Judging from the titles, madness seems the most persistent indication, as in Mia Lundin's *Female Brain Gone Insane*, Sheryl Currentz and Cindy Singer's *A Strange Period: Insights into the Bizarre Experiences of Perimenopausal Women*, and Sandra Tsing Loh's *The Madwoman in the Volvo*. What is noticeable in these menopausal musings is both a sense of humour and a desire to give testimonies from themselves and their clients— testimonies that can be helpful in assessing the visibility of one's own symptoms in crossing the void.

Loh quite rightly secures menopausal "madness" among any number of other mid-life calamities that she faced in her "year of raging hormones" (274): her split from her husband, her estrangement from her teenage children, or her extramarital affair with Mr. X. The "Volvo" (read "vulva") of the title becomes a menopausal "family friend," an old car that finally "is allowed to remain who she is" (274).

Loh presented her autobiographical critique on stage at the South Coast Repertory Theater in 2016. The reviewer for the *Los Angeles Times* was slightly annoyed by Loh's digressions but deemed the performance commendable for its "witty sociological commentary and its refusal to accept clichéd notions of biology as destiny" (McNulty).

In any survey of the current menopausal trends, one should not ignore the vivacious video performances of Menopause Barbie. This is the persona developed by Dr. Barbara Taylor, a nontypical gynecologist who, in a series of 127 (to date) ditzy videos, covers every imaginable topic having to do with the menopausal transition—from diet, to exercise, to psychological symptoms, to makeup, to makeovers, to a food guide for menopausal munchies—and covers them not in the drab white coat of the clinician but in flamboyant floppy hats and multicoloured string sundresses. The half-hour episodes, accessible from her *Menopause Taylor* website, are based in part on her 2008 self-published paperback: *Menopause: Your Management Your Way... Now and for the Rest of Your Life.*

The most valuable video tutorials from Taylor's collection for this chapter are #31, "Botanical and Herbal Estrogens," and #34, "Introduction to SERMS" (selective estrogen receptor modulators). In the latter, Barbie's estrogen replacement therapy tutorial is enhanced by plastic models of female organs and by other useful contraptions, such as vaginal inserts, which help to explain the risks and benefits of synthetic hormones. Although as a video doctor, she is not in the position to advocate for any of the prescription drugs, she cheerfully announces her motto: "Keep your vagina happy by getting enough estrogen." In #31, Menopause Barbie outlines the benefits and risks of "estrogen imposters," products derived from black cohosh and other botanical substances, which are nonhormonal but that can still be of great benefit to the breasts, the heart, the arteries, and the uterus. Ah, but here's the rub: Although this video has been revised since I first watched it, in an earlier version, Menopause Barbie, while assuming neutrality, encouraged the purchase of certain supplements available, without prescription, to her online patients when they clicked the desired merchandise into their empty shopping carts. As of 6 Feb. 2019, this tutorial offers information only on various herbs, compounds, and tinctures.

On an earlier iteration of Taylor's website, called *Menopause Barbie,* visitors were told that a Menopause Barbie doll was in the planning stage but not yet available for purchase. The doll has not materialized, but one wonders that if she had, would she have had flabby breasts and be prone to madness? Would she have been celebrated? Or would she have been a rubbery old blonde, a doll to dress and classify as one pleased, just another woman, her girlhood long gone, facing the void?

In sharp contrast with the first startling appearance of menstrual blood during puberty, the menopause, the final stage, is usually perceived as an absence, unmarked by the regularity and predictability of the menstrual cycle and filled with inconsistencies and contradictions. Although most menstrual celebrations are initiated by the presence of the bleeding that occurs at puberty, the menopausal absence has no parallel ceremony; it generally passes without celebration— invisible, defined only in retrospect. As I write in *Menstruation and Psychoanalysis*, "The menopause is the *end* of female genital bleeding, the once and future absence, when the threat of cultural contamination recedes" (4).

Puzzled by this absence, in mid-January of 2017, I sent an email query to a dozen or more postmenopausal feminists asking them if they had any experience with or knowledge of rituals surrounding the menopause. The answer was "No." So struck was I by the invisibility of the menopausal woman that my Baltimore friend Jo-Ann Pilardi, to whom this chapter is dedicated, offered to post an announcement on the list-serve of the National Women's Studies Association, describing my project and asking that they email me with their experiences, in person or in print, concerning menopausal rituals.

In response, Joan Starker sent me a copy of a poem, "Something to Look Forward To," in which Marge Piercy anticipates her own menopause in terms of ritual and celebration:

> I tell you I will secretly dance
> And pour out a cup of wine on the earth
> When time stops that leak permanently.

An eloquent personal response came from Lis Edna Valle-Ruiz, who described a rite of passage created by her close friends as Valle-Ruiz was preparing for a hysterectomy (or artificial menopause): "Two of us brought poems saying goodbye to the uterus, thanking it for the good things, asking for forgiveness for the not-so-good things, and letting go. Another person read scripture and shared some strengthening words. Two others shared prayers. One gave me a nest with an egg ... reminding us of our possibilities for being life-giving beings: that is the power of ritual." Jess Kilbourn sent me an account of a croning ceremony in honour of her spiritual leader: "Seventy women attended, making a corridor of their bodies and welcoming her to 'cronehood.' After that we offered her a vessel to put menstrual blood in that was collected from folks who were able to give blood from [the] community, and we made a tincture from it so that she is still able to access the power of menstrual blood for protection blessings."

Lee Lynch and Akia Woods have gathered together an astonishing assortment of menopausal blogs in their anthology *Off the Rag: Lesbians Writing on Menopause*. One of the longer entries describes a croning ceremony in which women congregated around an altar and brought pictures of female ancestors as well as jewelry, candles, and other ornaments; they danced and feasted in praise of two women experiencing the menopause. A key part of the ceremony involved re-entering the women's community and receiving a new identity and a new name—for example, "She-Who-Has-Gained-Control-Of-the-Inner-Fire" and "She-Who-is-The-Force-That-Moves-The-Moon" (Beckett and Wadley-Bailey, *Off the Rag* 73).

Artists and designers have also urged women to celebrate the menopause, either separately or collectively. The Instagram hashtag #menopauseart collates images from artists of various genres, creating a gallery without borders or bounds. One group, the Red Hot Mamas, advocates the artistic expression of the "change," referring their membership to an acrylic painting by Helen Redman titled *Hot Flashing* ("Embracing Menopause"). Coni Minneci, an artist from Western New York, transfers her perimenopausal experience of "abrupt changes, wet and fertile to dry" to the canvas in *Menopause Landscape*, a brilliantly barren oil and acrylic painting.

These and many other women have celebrated their aging through ritual, celebration, and self-affirmation. Sandra Tsing Loh wonders why menopausal women do not give each other baby showers. "We can register ourselves at As We Change and partake of festive party platters stocked with chocolates, wine and Ambien (not the generic kind, the good kind—because we're worth it!)" (243).

Although many women have defied the cultural norm by consciously acknowledging the change of life, such celebrations of menopausal control and power are rare. My own menopause slipped by—uncelebrated, unnoticed, and symptom free—during the peak of my academic career, when I was, ironically, nearing the end of my book on menstruation and psychoanalysis, totally unaware of what changes were occurring in my body.

Among the contemporary middle class, the postmenopausal woman is the gone girl, veiled in the cloak of invisibility and past her prime. This popular stereotype of the woman-after-menopause is marvellously characterized in the *Saturday Night Live* skit of October 1, 2016, in which presidential candidate Hillary Clinton, camouflaged in the youthful body of Kate McKinnon, somersaults onto the stage in a bright red pantsuit in defiance of her age, her position, and her reputed poor health.

The most lavishly staged tribute to the menopause, however, is *Menopause The Musical* by Jeanie Linders. The original show, first performed in Orlando, Florida, on March 28, 2001, has been viewed by a wide national and international audience. My husband, Ken Baldwin, and I saw the show on December 15, 2016, at Harrah's Casino in Las Vegas, Nevada, where there is an "open-ended" performance six nights a week.

Before the show, a woman came to our table offering promotional fans for sale for one dollar, with proceeds going to the National Breast Cancer Coalition, just the first of many puns on menopausal symptoms, in this case hot flashes. The seating was cabaret style, which particularly delighted us because near the end of the revue, the lead actress, Jacquelyn Holland-Wright, left the stage and straddled the man sitting adjacent to our table.

The plot of *Menopause the Musical* is minimal; it features four women who meet at Bloomingdale's, where they fight over a piece of lingerie. The thrill is in what follows: the music, the dance, and the solidarity as these women gradually unleash their shared biology. It is inexplicable that Sandra Tsing Loh should dismiss *Menopause The Musical* in a single paragraph, deriding it for its cheap plot and its minimal script: "nothing more than parodies of pop hits from the fifties and sixties, rewritten in the vernacular of svitzing and bloating" (50-51). If Loh saw the show at all, she may perhaps be alluding to amateur performances by touring companies in Kalamazoo, Michigan or Bismarck, North Dakota, but hardly to the award-winning Vegas revue, which has consistently thrilled its audiences with its songs, costumes, and intensity.

The major problem with *Menopause The Musical* lies not in its performances but in its sponsorship. Embedded in each program is a coupon distributed by Estroven, the co-sponsor of the production, asking the name, address, birthday, and email address for anyone who is experiencing "(pre)menopausal symptoms" or who has "purchased over-the-counter menopause supplements in the last year" ("Program Notes"). The coupon also asks, for some curious reason, "What hotel are you staying at?" Page eight of the program features a glossy advertisement for Estroven.

It is apparent that if the original purpose of *Menopause the Musical* was to entertain and to delight, it also had the additional incentive to sell—not only to sell Estroven and the three other helpful drugs (Zoloft, Paxil, and Prozac) praised in the song "Thank You, Doctor" (*Songbook* 21) but also to sell those women who have never experienced hot flashes or bloating the idea that there is something wrong with them.

Linders's innovative lyrics have a cohesion that goes beyond the song, the dance, and the message. The opening theme of *Menopause The Musical*, which appropriately mimics Aretha Franklin's "Chain of Fools," introduces the theme of madness: "For five long years, I thought I'm losing my mind/but I found out, No, it's just a part of the change" ("Songbook" 5). Other songs emphasize the madness theme, as in this echo of Marvin Gaye: "I heard it through the grapevine/And I'm just about to lose my mind" ("Songbook" 7). My favourite song parrots the hit recorded by the Platters in 1955, "The Great Pretender": "Oh—oh yes I'm the great pretender/Pretending that I'm doing well/My mind goes void, then I get annoyed/My brain skips, but no one can tell" ("Songbook" 19).

The women are stereotypically overweight, puffin', needing exercise, wanting makeovers, wanting estrogen. Then comes an amazing shift, announced by the song "Good Vibrations" (*Songbook* 35). They go shopping, not for lingerie, but for vibrators. It is hilarious to see the meek Iowa housewife in the pink suit, played by Lori Legacy, march across the stage, transformed by her huge pink vibrator while the Tina Turner look-a-like burlesques: "What's love got to do, got to do with it?" ("Songbook" 37). With mics in hand, the cast sings "Only You," a tribute to good vibrations, dildos, and to another Platters first: "Only you and you alone can thrill me like you do/Forget my man, for now it's only you" ("Songbook" 39). The only lyric that remains virtually unchanged is Patti LaBelle's upbeat, self-affirmative 1984 ballad "New Attitude" ("Songbook" 40-41).

The climax of the Vegas revue is a ladies' version of YMCA called "This Is Your Day" (*Songbook*, 43), when willing participants from the audience are invited to do a line kick in celebration of the menopause. One of my greatest moments in the last thirty years was to drag myself on to the stage, without falling, and to link arms with Lisa Mack, the "What's Love Got to Do with It" performer. Women attending regional productions have reported similar pleasure in their close encounters with the *Menopause* cast (Lipson).

Performers and creators, from Menopause Barbie to the practicing crones to Jeanie Linders to the entire cast of *Menopause The Musical*, to every gone girl who has rescued the end of her cycle from invisibility and exposed it to the public eye—this is their day, their grand finale, their last hurrah.

So, "Girlfriend, are you listenin' to me.... This is Your Day!/Join us and sing it/This is Your Day" ("Songbook" 43).

Acknowledgements

Mary Jane Lupton thanks Jo-Ann Pilardi for posting the request for information on menopause and ritual on WMST-L on January 20, 2017. The following women responded: Louise Bernikov; Margaret Blanchard; Jess Kilbourn; Shirley Perry; Joan Starker; Emily Toth; Lis Valle-Ruiz; and Judy Waldman. She thanks Crystal Hardin of Cape May, NJ, for loaning her the CD and the *Songbook* for *Menstruation The Musical*.

Works Cited

Beckett, Judith E., and Paij Wadley-Bailey. "Two Old Maids." *Off the Rag: Lesbians Writing on Menopause*, edited by Lee Lynch and Akia Woods, Victoria, 1996, pp. 68-74.

Clifton, Lucille. *The Collected Poems of Lucille Clifton 1965-2010*, edited by Kevin Young and Michael S. Glaser, BOA Editions, 2012.

Currentz, Sheryl, and Singer, Cindy. *A Strange Period: Insights into the Bizarre Experiences of Perimenopausal Women.* iUniverse, 2011.

Delaney, Janice, Mary Jane Lupton, and Emily Toth. *The Curse: A Cultural History of Menstruation.* Illinois University Press, 1988.

Dillaway, Heather E., and Jean Burton. "'Not Done Yet?!' Women Discuss the 'End' of Menopause." *Women's Studies*, vol. 40, no. 2, 2011, pp. 149-76.

"Estring." *Estring*, www.estring.com/vaginal-atrophy-relief. Accessed 30 Jan. 2019.

Fenton, Siobhan. "Menopause reversed as scientists successfully 'rejuvenate women's ovaries.'" *The New Scientist*, 21 July 2016, www. independent.co.uk/life-style/health-and-families/health-news/ scientists-successfully-reverse-menopause-by-rejuvenating-womens -ovaries-a7147981.html. Accessed 2 Jan. 2017.

Lipson, Karin. "That Familiar Play-Along Celebration of Menopause." *The New York Times*, 30 July 2010, www.nytimes.com/2010/08/01/ nyregion/01theatli.html. Accessed 11 Jan 2017.

Loh, Sandra Tsing. *The Madwoman in the Volvo*. Norton, 2014.

Lundin, Mia. *Female Brain Gone Insane*. Health Communications, 2009.

Lupton Mary Jane. *Elizabeth Barrett Browning*. Baltimore: Feminist Press, 1972.

Lupton Mary Jane. *Lucille Clifton: Her Life and Letters*. Westport, CT: Praeger, 2006.

Lupton Mary Jane. *Menstruation and Psychoanalysis*. Illinois University Press 1993.

McNulty, Charles. "Critic's Choice: 'The Madwoman in the Volvo' Offers a Comic Romp through a Midlife Crisis." 12 Jan. 2016, www. latimes.com/entertainment/arts/la-et-cm-madwoman-volvo-play-review-20160112-column.html. Accessed 30 Jan. 2017.

Minnechi, Coni. "Menopause Landscape." *The Art of Menstruation at the Museum of Menstruation and Women's Health*, www.mum.org/ pausminn.htm. Accessed 30 Jan. 2019.

Menopause: The Musical. "Program Notes." GFOUR Productions, 1916.

Menopause: The Musical. "The Songbook." GFOUR Productions, www. GFourProductions.com. Accessed 30 Jan. 2019.

Menopause: The Musical. Audio Disk. *Discogs*. www.discogs.com/ Various-Menopause-The-Musical/release/8456293. Accessed 30 Jan. 2019.

Northrup, Christiane, M.D. *The Wisdom of Menopause*. Bantam, 2012.

"Premarin." Advertisement. Pfizer, PP-PEM-USA-0162-01, 2016. *People*, 3 Jan. 2017.

Red Hot Mamas. "Embracing Menopause." *Red Hot Mamas*, 26 May 2010, redhotmamas.org/embracing-menopause/. Accessed 6 Feb. 2019.

Sexton, Anne. "Menstruation at Forty." *Poem Hunter*, www.poem hunter.com/best-poems/anne-sexton/menstruation-at-forty/. Accessed Sept. 21, 2017.

Taylor, Barbara D. *Menopause: Your Management Your Way... Now and for the Rest of Your Life.* Self-published, 2008.

Taylor, Barbara D. *Menopause Taylor*, menopausetaylor.me/. Accessed 6 Feb. 2019.

Taylor, Barbara D. "Botanical and Herbal Estrogens for Menopause —31." *YouTube*, 3 Jan. 2017, www.youtube.com/watch?v=FK53 MFgAdgM. Accessed 6 Feb. 2019.

Taylor, Barbara D. "Introduction to SERMs for Menopause—34." *Menopause Taylor.* Jan. 24, 2017, www.youtube.com/watch?v=tq BP6Xp3DLY. Accessed 6 Feb. 2019.

Wilson, Robert A. *Feminine Forever.* M. Evans, 1966.

Chapter 3

Myths and Misconceptions: Migrant and Refugee Women's Constructions and Experiences of Menopause

Jane Ussher, Alexandra Hawkey, and Janette Perz

Constructing Menopause as a Deficiency Disease

It is a bitter irony: Menstruation is positioned as a woman's curse within cultural and biomedical discourse (Kissling), yet the end of the reproductive years does not bring a reprieve from women being positioned as mad, moody, or vulnerable because of the womb (Ussher 92). In the nineteenth century, menopause was positioned as a time of reproductive crisis, with the central nervous system in disarray; thus, menopause was "universally admitted to be a critical and dangerous time for women" (Tilt 15). Twentieth-century medicine continued this pathologizing discourse through establishing the myth of menopausal deficiency disease as a medical truth and normalizing the practice of a medically managed midlife through hormonal replacement therapy (HRT) (Wilson 43). The menopausal woman was positioned as inherently debilitated by the "deficiency" of her aging body, her "senile" ovaries described by one medical text as a "shrunken and puckered organ, containing few if any follicles" (Netter 34), which resulted in the "death of womanhood" (Wilson 16).

The association between the biological materiality of menopause[1] and psychological disturbance is central to pathologizing discourse and practice. Robert Wilson, who first advocated HRT in 1966 as a prophylactic medication for all women at midlife, declared, "Low spirits, sadness or despondency are common symptoms around the menopause and are considered to be caused by a lack of oestrogen" (36). This view has continued within contemporary biomedical pronouncements (Joffe and Bromberger 241; Steiner, Dunn, and Born 67) and has been perpetuated in self-help information for perimenopausal women, who are informed that they may "suffer physical and psychological turmoil which makes this time a stormy passage" (Coupland and Williams 443).

Researchers have proclaimed that depression experienced by women who are menopausal is caused by changing hormonal levels, which affects hypothalamic functioning, neuropeptides and neurotransmitters, or the "synchrony or coherence between components of the circadian system" (Deeks 19). However, there is no clear evidence that the body causes women's physical or psychological distress during the menopausal transition. Although women are more likely to experience depression than men at any time in the lifecycle (Ussher 17), the rates of depression actually fall with age; thus, the notion of the menopausal woman being in a state of psychological turmoil is a myth. For example, in Australia, the highest rates of depression are found in women aged eighteen to twenty-four (Australian Bureau of Statistics), with the majority of women aged forty-five to fifty-five reporting that they experience positive mental health (Dennerstein 146). Similarly, in research examining women aged forty to fifty-nine living in New York, the majority reported feeling happy (McQuaide 21), with the factors predicting wellbeing including higher income as well as having a close group of friends, good health, high self-esteem, goals for the future, and positive feelings about appearance. These findings suggest that it is social context and women's negotiation of midlife and perimenopausal changes that lead to, or protect against, depression, not the deficient menopausal body (Ussher 53).

The Cultural Context of Menopause

Biological and sociocultural factors interact to modulate the construction and experience of embodied and psychological changes experienced at midlife (Bitzer and Alder 41). In this vein, cross-cultural research has provided compelling evidence that the meaning of menopause within specific cultural contexts can influence experience of symptoms (Kaufert and Syrotuik 174). For example, in a study comparing depression at midlife in North American and Japanese women, Nancy Avis and colleagues report that there were much lower rates in the Japanese group, which reflects the more positive constructions of women's aging in Japan, where menopause is positioned as a normal life transition (2014). In a more recent study comparing constructions and experiences of menopause in Australia and Laos, Australian women reported higher rates of depression as well as fears associated with aging, weight gain, and cancer—fears not reported by Laotian women, who understood menopause as a positive event (Sayakhot, Vincent, and Teede 1306).

Japanese and Laotian women have also been reported to be less likely than Caucasian women to report vasomotor symptoms, such as hot flushes, or to report embarrassment or distress if they do experience a hot flush during the menopausal transition (Lock 313; Sayakhot, Vincent, and Teede 1306). Within Western biomedical discourse, such symptoms are unequivocally linked to changes in estrogen levels and have been positioned as a factor in menopausal depression (Natari et al. 109). However, men also experience hot flushes (and other vasomotor symptoms) at midlife (Calvaresi and Bryan 225), and the reporting of hot flushes varies widely across cultures, ranging from 0 per cent of Mayan women (Beyene 46) to 5 per cent of Indonesian women (Haines et al. 264), and to 80 per cent of Dutch women (Dennerstein 151). Asian women from a range of cultural backgrounds (Haines et al. 270; Loh et al. 169), and their physicians (Lock, 314), have been reported to focus on bodily aches and pains as symptoms of menopause rather than hot flushes or other vasomotor symptoms. This finding demonstrates that signs of illness, and the symptom cluster we adopt, are culturally located rather than a simple reflection of embodied experiences.

The way in which embodied changes are constructed and experienced by individual women during the menopausal transition will determine the degree to which these changes are distressing and whether such changes are positioned as menopausal symptoms (Hunter 261; Koster and Garde 52). In the West, expectations of menopause have been found to be much more negative than the reality (Hunter and O'Dea 204), with women repeatedly reporting surprise and relief that their experiences do not match the pessimistic picture perpetuated by biomedical and cultural discourses (Stephens 654). Indeed, in research with Australian women, the majority reported that they were not troubled by their experience of vasomotor or somatic changes at midlife (Calvaresi and Bryan 225), with negative attitudes to menopause and aging related to women's positioning of body changes as "symptomatology" (Dennerstein 153). Equally, whereas some women will accept changes in fat distribution postmenopause, others will feel out of control in their bodies and, by extension, in their lives (Deeks 22; Perz and Ussher 296).

Cultural constructions of menopause, internalized by women, thus play a significant part in creating negative expectations and experiences and influencing menopausal management (Lock; Hall, Berry, and Matsumura). Little is known, however, about the meaning of menopause for vulnerable groups of women, such as migrant and refugee women (Im and Meleis 85). Such women may need to negotiate contradictory meanings of menopause in their country of origin and their host country (Ussher et al. 1916); they are known to have limited access to sexual and reproductive health information and support (Mengesha, Dune, and Perz). In a study of Korean women who had migrated to the United States, these women reported menopause to be an ambivalent experience; it was associated not only with the end of womanhood, due to failing fertility, but also with an unspoken experience, stemming from cultural taboos about talking about menstruation and sexuality (Im and Meleis 97). In the remainder of this chapter, we examine constructions of menopause in migrant and refugee women living in Australia and Canada across a range of cultural backgrounds and present some of the findings of a recent research study we conducted.

Migrant and Refugee Women's Negotiation of Menopause Study Description

The detailed methodology of the study has been published elsewhere (Ussher et al.). In summary, we conducted eighty-four individual interviews and sixteen focus groups with eighty-five participants (total n=169) with women aged eighteen years and over (average age thirty-five), who had settled in Australia or Canada in the last ten years; these women had migrated from Afghanistan, Iraq, Somalia, South Sudan, Sudan, Sri Lanka (Tamil), India (Punjab), and varying South American countries. Women practiced a range of religions, including Islam,

Christianity, Sikhism, and Hinduism. All participants, except for one Latina woman, identified as being heterosexual. The majority of interviews (73 per cent, n=124) were conducted in the first language of the participants by community interviewers and focused on experiences across the reproductive lifecycle, including menstruation, menopause, contraception, and sexual health. In our analysis, we adopted a material-discursive-intrapsychic theoretical approach (Ussher 106), which recognizes the materiality of the body, as well as other aspects of experience, but conceptualizes this materiality as always mediated by discourse, culture, and psychological negotiation. This viewpoint emphasizes how understandings of menopause and the menopausal body are influenced by cultural norms and discourses, which constitute bodily feelings and behaviours and which come to "constitute the phenomenology of embodiment" (Tolman, Bowman, and Fahs 761). In the accounts below, we use pseudonyms, age (or FG [focus group interview]), and cultural group when presenting quotes from women. We found no notable differences across women living in Canada or Australia.

Menopause as the Age of Despair

Across all cultural groups interviewed, menopause was discursively positioned in a negative manner and reflected hegemonic constructions of menopause in traditional patriarchal societies (Hall, Berry, and Matsumura 110). For instance, Sudanese participants told us that in their culture, menopause was described as "Sin Al Ya-iss," which translates to "age of despair" (Nasima, forty-three, Iraqi). Following menopause, a "woman is not as she was before" (FG, Sudanese) because menopause causes "discomfort just like the menstruation" (FG, Latina). Although menarche and menstruation were predominantly constructed and experienced as shameful and disgusting, leading to concealment and regulation of the reproductive body (Hawkey et al.), many women positioned the materiality of menstrual blood as playing a purifying role, which rids a woman's body of toxins, and thus, once menstrual bleeding ceases, women are subject to poor health. As Darya (twenty-four, Afghani) told us, "Your period, it ejects a lot of toxins from your body ... it may not be a good thing when it dries up.... Some people say you need special care once it stops and your health starts to fail because of that." Similarly, Arifa (forty-eight, Iraqi) described she was not looking forward to menopause, as she imagines she "will be getting ill, and blood will be accumulated in [her] body," and, consequently, she will "not have any more energy" and would, therefore, "love" if her period were to stay. These accounts suggest that although women may appear to be resisting the discursive positioning of a woman's bleeding as a source of stigma (Johnston-Robledo and Chrisler), by focusing on the danger of the "dried up" womb, these women reinforce the positioning of the reproductive body as abject and a source of women's poor health. Such a sentiment is illustrated in the following comment: "I hear that the woman, when the menstruation stop, every year, she should go and check for cancer" (FG, Sudanese).

Most women were premenopausal at the time of the interview and described a number of expected embodied changes during the menopausal transition, most of which were viewed negatively. For instance, Raana (forty-three, Iraqi) said, "I know the hormone will stop, and this will affect your bones and your health in general, so you'll either be exposed to maybe heart attack or to poor bone density." And Geet (thirty, Punjabi) told us: "[You] get irregular periods. Mood changes ... people get temperature changes quite frequently. Their body shape also changes. Their food habits change. So it's pretty much an extended lot of period the PMS." A Tamil focus group participant described menopause as "the body is very heat and mentally all the pressure, you know." Participants who had experienced, or were experiencing menopause, described it as a biological event with symptoms attributed to the material body. As Najiba (sixty-four, Iraqi) described: "I had [a] rash [and] feel depressed, older. Sometimes I feel my sexual life is finished, and I got very soft bones, always have back pain, hip pain. All this is the result of menopause." These accounts draw on a biomedical discourse, wherein menopause is positioned as a deficiency disease, and "raging hormones" (Vines 192) are the root of women's disembodiment.

In addition to material changes to the body, premenopausal women also discussed at length expected changes in relation to their intrapsychic wellbeing. Nasima (forty-three, Iraqi) said: "I would not like to get menopause. I believe losing my period will negatively affect my psyche." And an Iraqi focus group member told us that "After menstruation stops, the body becomes, sick and the woman suffers depression." Given these are the expected psychological changes, it is not surprising that a number of women attributed the negative changes with their midlife mood to the menopausal transition, as the following account demonstrates: "For me, there has been a lot of big changes in mood for the past year. I've had a lot of sort of mood frictions. [I'm] very sad lately, depressed. I just want to sit and cry more often, and [I'm] upset" (FG, Afghani).

As described by Hawkey, Ussher, and Perz, migrant and refugee women often described coming from cultural backgrounds in which a woman's fertility is highly regarded. In this vein, the end of fertility at menopause was considered a further factor in negatively viewing this transition. As Fahmo (twenty, Somali) described: "I think there is a negative stigma that follows the word 'menopause' around. Yeah, they [say] like 'oh, she is not able to give birth anymore. She is useless.'" As a consequence of the loss of fertility, some women described men leaving their wives: "I think for us, the culture, the people don't like [menopause] ... because when they're in menopause time, I think the husband thinks, 'Ah, she is in menopause. I think I might go back to marrying again, I will have another one.' Things like that" (Joyce, forty-five, South Sudanese). Menopause was also stigmatized as a life transition because it was associated with aging. For example, Nadiya said, "I've become like an aged person, so it [menopause] is just hidden" (Nadiya, seventy, Iraqi), and a focus group member from Sudan said that with menopause, a "woman feels that she is now old" and "she may suffer laziness, some psychological symptoms."

These accounts illustrate the ways in which negative social constructions of menopause, and of women's aging, may negatively affect a woman's expectations, as well as her actual experience of, the physical and psychological changes related to the menopausal transition.

A Discourse of Silence and Secrecy

Across all cultural groups, a discourse of silence and secrecy resulted in many women having limited knowledge in relation to menopause, which potentially contributed to their negative expectations and experiences of psychological and embodied changes during this time. Participants told us that they had come from cultural contexts in which "anything sexually related was a taboo subject" (Homa, forty, Afghani). As described by Ussher et al., such silence and secrecy were in relation not only to menopause but also to broader aspects of women's sexual and reproductive health, including menarche and menstruation, contraception, sexual desire, and sexual pain in marriage (1908). For instance, women described that they were "a little bit shy" (Raana, forty-two, Iraqi) about discussing menstruation with their daughters: "It is sham[ful] to talk about sex with anyone in my culture and I feel embarrassed to talk about it" (Hooria, thirty-five, Sudanese). Another participant also said that "no one would talk to another person [about contraception]" (Akeck, 31, Sudanese). Similarly, regarding menopause, women described that they had nobody to talk to: "In our culture, I don't think people will talk about it" (Aameeka, forty, Tamil). Talking about menopause was silenced because other people "think if they speak it means I am aged; so they don't speak it" (Nadiya, seventy, Iraqi). These accounts are similar to those of Korean migrant women living in the United States (Im and Meleis) and Canada (Elliott, Berman, and Kim), where women experienced menopause alone because sexual and reproductive health was rarely talked about and menopause was a taboo subject even within families.

As a consequence of this silence and secrecy, many women disclosed having a lack of accurate knowledge surrounding menopause, with women aged thirty to fifty admitting that they knew nothing about it. Aameeka (forty, Tamil), for example, said: "I don't know how that works. If it is periods, okay, you know, every month you bleed and stuff like that, but menopause, how does it work? I don't know that." And Azita (thirty-seven, Afghani) said: "I don't know what is going to happen.... I don't have any information about this" (Azita). This limited knowledge allowed myths and misconceptions in relation to menopause and women's reproductive bodies to remain unchallenged. For example, one woman said, "I heard that if you remove your uterus, your eyesight will be affected" (FG, Afghani). Another participant disclosed that she "met one lady who is nearly fifty years [old].... she said, 'I don't want to talk to you ...don't disturb me,' [but] it is okay. I understand because she is that time [menopause]." The absence of a possibility to discuss, understand, and normalize possible changes during menopause means that many women do not have a framework to challenge the cultural construction of menopause as an age of despair.

Menopause as a Life Stage—or When Life Starts

Across cultural groups, however, a number of women did challenge negative constructions or experiences of menopause; they resisted the positioning of the menopausal woman as abject and menopause as a deficiency disease. For some women, this resistance was facilitated by migration as well as an awareness of alternative discourses (Coupland and Williams), in which midlife and menopause are viewed as a time when life starts for women.

It was following migration they had a new outlook towards menopause: "I used to hear about menopause, when the menstruation stops, the woman feels that her age is now come to an end, and she suffered depression, but here in Canada, they don't think [this] about menopause. After menopause, life starts" (FG, Iraqi). A number of participants also described menopause as just "another stage" (Raana, forty-three, Iraqi) and a "natural transition many women were curious about." Ariana, (forty, Latina), said the following: "I think it is the end of the reproductive stage as a woman and then it is the beginning of the second stage. For now, I don't have worries, for now I have only curiosity, but I guess my feelings in regards to menopause and my point of view are going to be changing as the time is getting closer. For now, I have only curiosity."

At the same time, a number of women who were experiencing embodied or psychological changes during the menopausal transition normalized such changes and looked to natural means of coping: "I can feel, sometimes feel stress, but it's okay, normal, and even [the doctor] asks me, if you have tablets [hormones] to keep it [menopause], I don't want to, I just go for natural things and that's it, yeah" (Nasira, 52, Iraqi). Natural remedies for menopausal change were also commonly used by Korean migrants living in Canada (Hall, Berry, and Matsumura 384), demonstrating that women find means of coping that are available and acceptable within their own cultural context.

A number of women adopted counternarratives to the positioning of the cessation of monthly menstrual periods and decline in fertility associated with menopause as negative. As Geet (thirty, Punjabi) said, "Once I have kids, I just want to get it over and done with. Then I can enjoy life without having to worry about these monthly cramps, which is—it [menopause] might be a good blessing in disguise, if there is such a thing." In a similar vein, a Latina focus group participant said: "I think if you stop bleeding, I think that's something good that happens to us.

I look forward to have the menopause because I am not going to ... have these painful menstruation cycles." Furthermore, Ariana (forty, Latina) stated that she viewed menopause in a positive light as she would no longer need to worry about becoming pregnant: "I am forty, so I know that it is difficult for me to get pregnant, so I feel very relieved and very lucky because I don't have to worry about that, and I can finally enjoy sex without being worried that I am going to get pregnant. This is one of the best things about aging."

Many women also resisted a discourse of silence and secrecy associated with menopause, and the subsequent negative implications for health and wellbeing, by obtaining information about the expected changes during this transition. Some gained information through mothers and friends. For example, Ariana (forty, Latina) "I don't have much information. I only have like general information and that is through my interaction and conversations of women that are already with the menopause, or are starting to experience the beginning of the menopause." Other women looked for information on the internet or talked to work colleagues who were not constrained by cultural taboos. As Aameeka (forty, Tamil) said: "These days, I am trying to go through the internet and check [for menopause information]. I'm trying because I feel that I am in that stage now. Yeah...I want to talk about it too. I have a work colleague. She is very open minded, and she talks about it, so I'm trying to talk to her and find out." Similarly, Suz (forty-two, South Sudanese) said: "I don't know. I don't know. I'm hearing that [menopause] on the television. Like yesterday, they say menopause.... I've got to go to the doctor and ask about that. I don't know what that means. It has been worrying me. That's why I want to find out."

These accounts suggest that it is important for migrant and refugee women to have access to information to not only support their understanding of menopause as a normal life transition but also to counter negative cultural discourse associated with the reproductive body that may be present in their communities (Hall, Berry, and Matsumura 114).

Conclusion

These accounts of migrant and refugee women provide insight into the commonalities and differences in constructions and experiences of menopause across a range of cultural contexts. Negative constructions of menopause, associated with silence and secrecy, were evident across all cultural groups, which has implications for women's positioning and experience of menopausal change and embodiment. However, resistance to negative discourse was also evident, which was primarily associated with education and more open communication about menopausal change, suggesting that education and health information can help to affirm aspects of menopause. As a result, women may feel more positively about changes they experience during this transition.

There are a number of practical implications of these findings for service providers. The advancement of migrant and refugee women's sexual and reproductive rights requires a combination of system improvements and services that benefit women (Sen and Govender 230). This includes acknowledging the specific needs of migrant and refugee women and the production of culturally safe health promotion strategies as well as sexual and reproductive health resources. Sexual and reproductive health promotion needs to be a key part of early resettlement for migrant and refugee women (McMichael and Gifford 230) and should include the provision of information on perimenopause and menopause for community workers to provide to these women (Ussher et al. 1917). When providing education about menopause, healthcare professionals and community workers should first assess cultural beliefs and knowledge of those they seek to support while respecting those beliefs and assessing whether those women, in fact, desire such knowledge and intervention (Hall, Berry, and Matsumura 115). Menopause does not have to be constructed or experienced as a negative or fearful experience. Breaking the silence through communication and education and providing appropriate support for those women who do report distress can serve to challenge negative discourses and practices. Furthermore, this can facilitate the production of more positive and enabling cultural constructions of menopausal embodiment.

Endnotes

1. While acknowledging the established clinical distinction between perimenopause (the transitional period to menopause) and meno-pause (the time of life that begins one year past the last menstrual period), we at times in this paper use the term "menopause" inter-changeably or collectively to refer to perimenopause, menopause,

and/or menopausal transition. This reflects how these terms are used in the research we cite and how the women we interviewed talked about the menopausal experience.

Works Cited

Australian Bureau of Statistics. "National Survey of Mental Health and Wellbeing: Summary of Results, 2007." *ABS*, 2008, www.abs.gov.au/ausstats/abs@.nsf/productsbytitle/3F8A5DFCBECAD9C0CA2568A900139380?OpenDocument, Accessed 28 Nov. 2018.

Avis, Nancy, et al. "The Evolution of Menopause Symptoms." *International Practice and Research*, vol. 7, no. 1, 1993, pp. 17-32.

Beyene, Yewoubdar. "Cultural Significance and Physiological Manifestations of Menopause: A Biocultural Analysis." *Culture, Medicine and Psychiatry*, vol. 10, no. 1, 1986, pp. 46-71.

Bitzer, J., and J. Alder. "Cultural and Ethnic Influences on the Menopause Transition." *Key Issues in Mental Health*, vol. 175, 2009, pp. 41-49.

Calvaresi, Eva, and Janet Bryan. "Symptom Experience in Australian Men and Women at Midlife." *Maturitas*, vol. 44, no. 3, 2003, pp. 225-36.

Coupland, Justine, and Angie Williams. "Conflicting Discourses, Shifting Ideologies: Pharmaceutical, 'Alternative,' and Feminist Emancipatory Texts on the Menopause." *Discourse and Society*, vol. 13, no. 4, 2002, pp. 419-45.

Deeks, Amanda A. "Psychological Aspects of Menopause Management." *Best Practice and Research in Clinical Endocrinology and Metabolism*, vol. 17, no. 1, 2003, pp. 17-31.

Dennerstein, Lorraine. "Well-Being, Symptoms and the Menopausal Transition." *Maturitas*, vol. 23, no. 3, 1996, pp. 147-57.

Elliott, Janice, Helene Berman, and Sue Kim. "A Critical Ethnography of Korean Canadian Women's Menopause Experience." *Health Care for Women International*, vol. 23, no. 4, 2002, pp. 377-88.

Haines, Christopher J., et al. "Prevalence of Menopausal Symptoms in Different Ethnic Groups of Asian Women and Responsiveness to Therapy with Three Doses of Conjugated Estrogens/Medroxyprogesterone Acetate: The Pan-Asia Menopause (PAM) Study." *Maturitas*, vol. 52, no. 3, 2005, pp. 264-76.

Hall, Lisa, Judith Berry, and Geraldine Matsumura. "Meanings of Menopause: Cultural Influences on Perception and Management of Menopause." *Journal of Holistic Nursing*, vol. 25, no. 2, 2007, pp. 106-18.

Hawkey, A., J., M. Ussher, and J. Perz. "'If You Don't Have a Baby, You Can't Be in Our Culture': Migrant and Refugee Women's Exper-iences and Constructions of Fertility and Fertility Control." *Women's Reproductive Health*. Forthcoming.

Hawkey, A. J., et al. "Experiences and Constructions of Menarche and Menstruation among Migrant and Refugee Women." *Qualitative Health Research*, vol. 27, no. 10, 2017, pp. 1473-90.

Hunter, Myra. "Bio-Psycho-Socio-Cultural Perspectives on Meno-pause." *Best Practice & Research Clinical Obstetrics & Gynaecology*, vol. 21, no. 2, 2007, pp. 261-74.

Hunter, Myra, and Irene O'Dea. "Menopause: Body Changes and Multiple Meanings." *Body Talk: The Material and Discursive Construction of Sexuality, Madness and Reproduction*, edited by J. M. Ussher, Routledge, 1997, pp. 199-222.

Im, Eun-Ok, and Afaf Ibrahim Meleis. "Meanings of Menopause to Korean Immigrant Women." *Western Journal of Nursing Research*, vol. 22, no. 1, 2000, pp. 84-102.

Joffe, H., and J. T. Bromberger. "Shifting Paradigms about Hormonal Risk Factors for Postmenopausal Depression: Age at Menopause as an Indicator of Cumulative Lifetime Exposure to Female Reproductive Hormones." *JAMA Psychiatry*, vol. 73, no. 2, 2016, pp. 111-12.

Johnston-Robledo, Ingrid, and Joan C. Chrisler. "The Menstrual Mark: Menstruation as Social Stigma." *Sex Roles*, vol. 68, no. 1-2, 2013, pp. 9-18.

Kaufert, P., and J. Syrotuik. "Symptom Reporting and the Menopause." *Social Science and Medicine*, vol. 184, 1981, pp. 173-84.

Kissling, E. A. *Capitalizing on the Curse: The Business of Menstruation*. Lynne Rienner Publishers, 2006.

Koster, A., and K. Garde. "Sexual Desire and Menopausal Development. A Prospective Study of Danish Women Born in 1936." *Maturitas*, vol. 16, 1993, pp. 49-60.

Lock, M. "Menopause in Cultural Context." *Experimental Gerontology*, vol. 29, no. 3-4, 1994, pp. 307-17.

Loh, Foo-Hoe, et al. "The Age of Menopause and the Menopause Transition in a Multiracial Population: A Nation-Wide Singapore Study." *Maturitas*, vol. 52, no. 3, 2005, pp. 169-80.

McMichael, Celia, and Sandra Gifford. "'It Is Good to Know Now... before It's Too Late': Promoting Sexual Health Literacy amongst Resettled Young People with Refugee Backgrounds." *Sexuality & Culture*, vol. 13, no. 4, 2009, pp. 218-36.

McQuaide, Sharon. "Women at Midlife." *Social Work*, vol. 43, no. 1, 1998, pp. 21-31.

Mengesha, Zelalem Birhanu, Tinashe Dune, and Janette Perz. "Culturally and Linguistically Diverse Women's Views and Experiences of Accessing Sexual and Reproductive Health Care in Australia: A Systematic Review." *Sexual Health*, vol. 13, no. 4, 2016, pp. 299-310.

Natari, R. B., et al. "The Bidirectional Relationship between Vasomotor Symptoms and Depression across the Menopausal Transition: A Systematic Review of Longitudinal Studies." *Menopause*, vol. 25, no. 1, 2018, pp. 109-20.

Netter, F. H. *A Compilation of Paintings on the Normal and Pathological Anatomy of the Reproductive System*, vol. 2. Ciba, 1965.

Perz, J., and J. M. Ussher. "The Horror of this Living Decay: Women's Negotiation and Resistance of Medical Discourses around Menopause and Midlife." *Women's Studies International Forum*, vol. 31, 2008, pp. 293-99.

Sayakhot, P., A. Vincent, and H. Teede. "Cross-Cultural Study: Experience, Understanding of Menopause, and Related Therapies in Australian and Laotian Women." *Menopause*, vol. 19, no. 12, 2012, pp. 1300-08.

Sen, Gita, and Veloshnee Govender. "Sexual and Reproductive Health and Rights in Changing Health Systems." *Global Public Health*, vol. 10, no. 2, 2015, pp. 228-42.

Steiner, M., E. Dunn, and L. Born. "Hormones and Mood: From Menarche to Menopause and Beyond." *Journal of Affective Disorders*, vol. 74, no. 1, 2003, pp. 67-83.

Stephens, Christine. "Women's Experience at the Time of Menopause: Accounting for Biological, Cultural and Psychological Embodiment." *Journal of Health Psychology*, vol. 6, no. 6, 2001, pp. 651-63.

Tilt, Edward John. *The Change of Life in Health and Disease. A Clinical Treatise on the Diseases of the Ganglionic Nervous System Incidental to Women at the Decline of Life*. Bermingham, 1882.

Tolman, D. L., C. P. Bowman, and B. Fahs. "Sexuality and Embodiment." *APA Handbook of Sexuality and Psychology: Vol. 1. Person-Based Approaches*, edited by D. L. Tolman and L. M. Diamond, American Psychological Association, 2014, pp. 759-804.

Ussher, J. M. *The Madness of Women: Myth and Experience*. Routledge, 2011.

Ussher, J. M., et al. "Negotiating Discourses of Shame, Secrecy, and Silence: Migrant and Refugee Women's Experiences of Sexual Embodiment." *Archives of Sexual Behavior*, vol. 46, no. 7, 2017, pp. 1901-21.

Vines, Gale. *Raging Hormones: Do They Rule Our Lives?* University of California Press, 1993.

Wilson, Robert. *Feminine Forever*. M. Evans, 1966.

Chapter 4

The SWAN Study: Gender, Race, Identity, and Menopause

Mindy Fried

Researcher as Study Participant

I sit opposite Lila, [1] the twenty-something research assistant. We're in a small treatment room located in a labyrinth of satellite offices of Massachusetts General Hospital. Lila is warm and professional as she greets me, one of hundreds of research subjects she invariably encounters each year. Before long, we discover that she earned her undergraduate degree from the same university where I earned my PhD in sociology. In fact, she even took classes with some of my favourite professors, and we determine that she might have attended a talk I gave on campus a number of years back. This is a nice icebreaker. But now, in this room, Lila is in the driver's seat. She has just finished asking me a series of questions about my health, lifestyle, and social networks. I will be there for a total of four hours by the time I complete the entire process, which includes a bone density scan and a few other tests that have been added to the study this year.

***

In 1996, right after I completed my PhD in sociology, I was randomly selected as one of 3,302 women from diverse racial/ethnic backgrounds to participate in a midlife women's health study called SWAN—or Study of Women's Health Across the Nation. [2] For over twenty years,

SWAN has been following study subjects as we transition through menopause. The aim is to help scientists, healthcare providers, and women in general better understand how the physical, biological, psychological, and social changes we experience during this process affect our health and quality of life.

Moreover, as members of the patient community being investigated, we benefit from the comprehensive data the study shares with its participants annually based on the physical exam component.

Having just completed my dissertation research at the time, I welcomed the opportunity to be a subject in someone else's study. But I felt particularly grateful to be a part of important research that had the prospect of influencing medical science. Although I knew I was agreeing to a longitudinal study, it did not occur to me at the time that I would have a decades-long relationship with this study or that I would be interviewed by at least fifteen young research assistants, as they cycled in and out of their jobs, many of them en route to medical school or other postgraduate work.

SWAN Study: Exploring the Impact of Race, Culture, and Ethnicity

At baseline—that is, when the study began—SWAN participants or subjects were all between forty-two and fifty-two years old. I was in my late forties. Together, we represented seven clinical study sites around the country, including my own city of Boston, two in California, and one each in Illinois, Michigan, New Jersey, and Pennsylvania. In Boston, the study has oversampled for African American women, and in other parts of the country, the study has oversampled for Asian and Latina women. Having data on such a diverse group of women throughout the United States has allowed researchers to explore critical questions about the impact of race, culture, and ethnicity on health outcomes of women as we age.

In fact, SWAN-affiliated researchers Robin Green and Nanette Santoro have found that most symptoms of menopausal women vary by ethnicity: "Vasomotor symptoms were more prevalent in African-American and Hispanic women and were also more common in women with greater BMI, challenging the widely held belief that obesity is protective against vasomotor symptoms" (127). They also found that vaginal dryness was present in between 30 and 40 per cent of SWAN participants at baseline and was most prevalent in Hispanic women (127). But even among Hispanic women, "symptoms varied by country of origin" (127). The researchers conclude that "acculturation appears to play a complex role in menopausal symptomatology" (127) and that ethnicity should be a factor when interpreting menopausal symptoms in women.

SWAN researchers Melissa Putman and colleagues have found that African American women have a lower risk of fracture than Caucasian women, which may be explained by "bone microarchitecture and density" differences ("Differences in Skeletal Microarchitecture" 2177) and that having Type 2 diabetes may negatively affect the bone architecture of African American women ("Defects in Cortical Microarchitecture" 673). By including an ethnically diverse sample, the SWAN study can compare the experiences of women from varied backgrounds, which has revealed important differences that should be of great benefit to healthcare practitioners.

Research Data Benefits Participants

As a study participant, I am grateful that SWAN researchers provide us with information about our health, and flag issues we should explore further. For example, I discovered a number of years ago that I had high cholesterol, something that runs in my family. Initially, I was referred to a specialist who asked me to take a very low dose of a statin drug. Because I am resistant to taking any medication, I negotiated with him to take a lower-than-therapeutic dose, which I continue to this day, and then made minor adjustments to my diet, adding more fibre. The upshot is that my cholesterol levels have reduced significantly, thanks to initial findings from SWAN.

Over ten years ago, I also discovered—through my bone density data from the SWAN study—that I had osteopenia, a lower than normal bone density, in my lower spine. Osteopenia is considered a risk factor for developing osteoporosis, a condition associated with porous, weak bones, which increases fracture risk. That knowledge prompted me to do more extensive research about my risk of fractures. I asked my primary care physician to refer me to a specialist, whom I saw for a decade. Ultimately, this physician prescribed Fosomax, a medication used to treat or prevent osteoporosis. Knowing there was some controversy around this drug gave me pause, but I trusted the specialist's knowledge and experience. Five years later, when she told me that new data had emerged about the rare but notable side effect of major thigh bone fractures (Black et al. 1761), I stopped taking the medication.

A few years ago, there was a funding hiatus for the study. I was having a tough year and barely noticed that I had not received the annual call to set up an appointment. But the following year, a letter arrived announcing that SWAN had been refunded and I would be contacted soon. I was thrilled the study was continuing in this age of budget cuts for basic science and social science research. Though relieved that my health was back on track, I felt somewhat regretful that my SWAN profile would not document my less than glowing year.

That said, it struck me that SWAN gave me a regular opportunity to reflect on my life's circumstances and to think about my gradual process of growing older. Responding to a set of questions read to me by an inexperienced but eager young research assistant was both invigorating and thought provoking. Not only did it make me think about my life and lifestyle, but it also got me thinking about the skewed dynamic between researchers and subjects. This was the first study in which I was a subject. Yet the young people interviewing me reminded me of undergraduate students I had taught or grad students I had hired as my own research assistants in the past. Although I was excited about being a participant in this study, I initially felt self-conscious sharing personal information. But over time, the dynamic shifted as I engaged the assistants in conversation about their experiences on this research project as well as more broadly about what they hoped for concerning their careers. Most were happy to talk, and I realized I had a positive role to play with these new researchers. I could support their learning process by being open and reflective in responding to their questions, and I could listen as they talked to me about their lives.

***

Lila, the research assistant, is trained to draw blood, and as she jabs me expertly with the needle I think, "Wow, she's not bad." We continue to chat, as she measures my waist and hips, clocks how fast I can walk down a narrow hallway, and how long I can balance in a variety of different positions. I'm feeling pretty cocky until we get to the cognitive test, which the study instituted about seven years ago. Even though I believe that my memory is still sharp, being quizzed by a young person is unnerving. I have taught sociology courses on aging, and I know the literature about memory and aging. I remind myself that anxiety affects memory, and I tell Lila that the test makes me anxious, and she says "Yeah, everyone hates it." That's only somewhat reassuring, but I appreciate her attempt to normalize my response. I do my best to respond to her questions. In one test, she reads a series of numbers and letters in random order such as: "a9w2x548lz." I am to reorder them, without aid of pen and paper, then say them back to her, first letters, then numbers like so: "alwxz24589." The longer the configurations of letters and numbers, the harder it is to recall them all. Lila also tells me a story about three children in a burning house being saved by a brave firefighter and then asks me to retell it with as many details as I remember. I will be told the same story when I return for my SWAN visit the following year. I will follow directions and retell the story, knowing that I'm acing it but still wondering if the use of the same story is intentional. I will ask the research assistant, but she will not respond.

***

In a paper about the impact of the menopause transition on memory, SWAN researchers Gail Greendale and colleague conclude the following:

> Consistent with transitioning women's perceived memory difficulties, perimenopause was associated with a decrement in cognitive performance, characterized by women not being able to learn as well as they had during premenopause. Improvement rebounded to premenopausal levels in postmenopause, suggesting that menopause transition-related cognitive difficulties may be time-limited. (1850)

Once again, data from the SWAN study provide relevant, and in this case reassuring, news regarding the normal aging process.

Gathering the SWANS

In the past couple of decades, the SWAN team has held a number of gatherings to bring Boston SWAN subjects together. It is inspiring to be in a room with hundreds of women with one thing in common: We are midlife women who are going through or have completed the menopause transition. What fun it is to talk about all the nuisances we are experiencing without feeling judged or worrying we might be boring someone.

The first gathering I attended offered workshops where experts answered our questions about sleep and the impact of hot flashes and suggested natural alternatives to hormone replacement therapy. One year, SWAN researchers organized an event that featured the brilliantly outspoken Jocelyn Elders, a former U.S. Surgeon General, who was a lightning rod for speaking her mind in support of legalizing marijuana, the distribution of contraceptives in schools, and even suggesting that masturbation might be a means of preventing young people from engaging in riskier forms of sexual activity. Sitting in a diverse crowd of midlife women in which I, as a white woman, was among the minority (since Boston oversampled African American women), I joined my fellow SWAN study subjects in cheering loudly for Elders. Having admired her for years, I was positively thrilled to be in her company.

***

Lila tells me about this year's gathering, which I unfortunately missed. I learn that one of the Boston-based principal investigators, Dr. Joel Finkelstein, is a serious art aficionado and at the last SWAN study gathering, he showed a series of paintings by an older woman. His message was that we can continue to grow and be creative as we age. When the interview is complete, Lila hands me my gift. In past years, it has been a cup or a small tote bag, marked with the graceful SWAN logo. But this year, it's a small box, the top graced with a floral design from this artist.

***

In the abstract of his 2014 application to the National Institutes of Health, Dr. Finkelstein concluded by saying:

> SWAN will fill important gaps in understanding the impact of the menopausal transition and mid-life aging on women's health and functioning in the postmenopausal years. Accordingly, it will provide useful information to guide clinical decisions in mid-life and beyond in women who have diverse life experiences and socioeconomic and racial/ethnic characteristics.

I'm thankful to be a part of this longitudinal study, to know that the aggregate data being collected reflect a diverse population of women, and that we are collectively contributing to scientific knowledge which can improve the lives of women as we age. Personally, I'm grateful for the positive benefits to my own health and wellness received over a twenty-five period as a SWAN participant.

Endnotes

1. The research assistant's name has been changed.
2. For more information about the SWAN study, please refer to the website: www.swanstudy.org.

Works Cited

Black, Dennis, et al, "Bisphosphonates and Fractures of the Sub-trochanteric or Diaphyseal Femur." *N Engl J Med,* vol. 362, no.19, 13 May 2010, pp.1761-71.

Finkelstein, Joel S., "Study of Women's Health Across the Nation—V." *National Institutes of Health,* grantome.com/grant/NIH/U01-AG012531-21A1#panel-comment. Accessed 6 Feb. 2019.

Green, Robin and Nanette Santoro, "Menopausal Symptoms and Ethnicity: The Study of Women Across the Nation." *Women's Health,* vol. 5, no. 2, Mar. 2009, pp.127-33.

Greendale, Gail A. et al, "Effects of the Menopause Transition and Hormone Use on Cognitive Performance in Midlife Women." *Neurology,* vol. 72 no. 21, 26 May 2009, pp. 1850-57.

Putman, Melissa S., et al. "Defects in Cortical Microarchitecture among African-American Women with Type 2 Diabetes." *Osteoporos Int.* vol. 26, no. 22, Feb. 2015, pp. 673-9. *National Center for Biotechnology Information,* www.ncbi.nlm.nih.gov/pubmed/2539 8431.

Putman, Melissa S., et al. "Differences in Skeletal Microarchitecture and Strength in African-American and White Women." *Journal of Bone and Mineral Research,* vol. 28, no. 10, Oct. 2013, pp. 2177-85.

Thurston, Rebecca, and Hadine Joffe. "Vasomotor Symptoms and Menopause: Findings from the Study of Women's Health Across the Nation." *Obstet Gynecol Clin North Am.* vol 38, no .32011 Sep. 2011, pp. 489-501.

Chapter 5

Slouching towards Menopause

Joanne Gilbert

I wasn't glad to see you
after almost a year of
living without you.
Your return, unbidden, unwanted
unhinged me
as I scrambled to find my
mooring,
sought what had become my
equilibrium.
The worst part was
not knowing whether
you would stay
or go
only to return
again.
I thought I was done with you
for good,
hoped I was,
made plans for a better life
without you,
anticipated the time
I could truly
celebrate
your departure,

dared not speak of
finality,
but prayed daily
that you would never
darken
my door.
And now,
the balance I'd begun
to achieve
recedes
as I struggle with
the chaos of
uncertainty.

—11/11/14

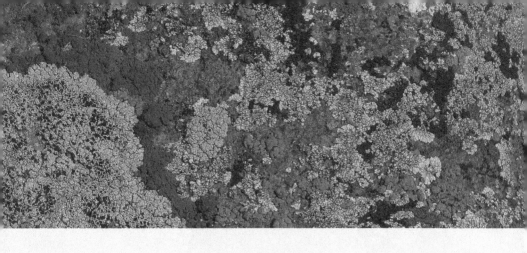

SECTION TWO

OUT OF STEP

Wherein the transition to menopause does
not happen at the age or in the way it is expected
to happen.

Chapter 6

Before Your Time: When Menopause Comes Too Soon

Evelina W. Sterling, Christine Eads, Starr Vuchetich, and Catherine M. Gordon

Traditionally, menopause is marked by the end of a woman's menstrual cycles. This experience is usually reserved for older woman and is characterized by an expected and natural transition into a new season of life. However, menstruation can stop at any age. Young women who experience a permanent cessation of menstruation do not share the same experiences—physically, emotionally, or socially—as older women. The reality is that women of varying ages experience menopause every day. For some, this change arrives too soon.

Early or premature menopause, premature ovarian failure, and primary ovarian insufficiency (POI) are all are terms commonly used to describe the condition that leads to menopause before the age of forty. The term "ovarian failure" is a misnomer, as it implies that women and their bodies have failed in some way. It also fails to capture the nuances of the condition: a progression, over time, of ovarian insufficiency. If the ovaries become insufficient, they no longer produce normal amounts of estrogen or release eggs regularly. However, not all women experience these changes in ovarian function in exactly the same way. A young woman's ovarian function can vary; it is not typically a case of her ovaries being absolutely on or absolutely off. For many women with ovarian insufficiency, ovaries still function but in an intermittent and unpredictable manner. This intermittent function can persist for decades. Some women experience irregular or occasional periods for several years, whereas others stop having periods altogether. As such, POI is the preferred term because it is more accurate and flexible in its description of what actually happens to ovarian function before the age of forty in women with this condition. (Welt 501). POI captures the continuum of impaired ovarian function rather than a specific endpoint of permanent ovarian function loss (Welt 501). By definition, POI has its onset before the age of forty and in some cases may occur as early as eleven years old (Covington et al. 140). Still considered rare, POI affects approximately 0.01 per cent of women under the age of twenty, 0.1 per cent of women under the age of thirty, and about 1 per cent of women overall (De Vos et al. 911). Though not as common in adolescents as young adults, POI significantly affects both the health and well-being of women at any age.

The perspectives of young women who experience early or premature menopause are often excluded from conversations about this reproductive transition. To provide these girls and young women with a voice and to develop a more inclusive understanding of menopause, we conducted in-depth, semistructured, IRB-approved interviews between 2008 and 2010 with fifty-two women from across the United States. Participants ranged in age from eighteen to fifty and all had stopped menstruating before the age of forty. Each interview was conducted either face to face or by telephone and lasted between sixty and ninety minutes. All interviews were digitally recorded and transcribed. These qualitative data were analyzed using a modified grounded theory approach to uncover significant themes that arose directly from the data. More information about the methodological details of this study can be found in the work of Evelina Sterling and Angie Best-Boss (2010). Data analyses illustrated the actual lived experiences that accompany the occurrence of early menopause (Sterling and Best-Boss 3).

In the spirit of qualitative research, we will include excerpts from interviews with women living with POI throughout this chapter. We will highlight quotes from a variety of women and offer additional context to explain their experiences, with a larger goal of contributing to the broad understanding of POI. Given both the complexity and uniqueness of living with POI, we think it is important to let the women in our study speak for themselves and only interpret their voices for the reader when necessary. We begin with a quote that illustrates some of the overall themes we highlight in this article. Elise, age thirty-six, focuses on the emotional and identity-based changes that occur once a woman receives a POI diagnosis:

> After the initial shock of finding out about going through meno-pause early, there are two ways people can go about living. They can be shy, ignore it, and beat themselves up for experiencing something that they can't control. Or they can accept themselves for how they are interpersonally, as well as biologically, and look beyond the stigma of having early menopause. I've chosen to live in the latter mode, and in doing so, I've received an overwhelming positive response from doctors, researchers, family, friends, and the community. I've found that the more information people know about going through menopause at a much younger age, the less scary it becomes and the more support they offer. Plus, I can focus more on adapting to my body's changes without focusing on what I lost.

So what's the big deal? Although individual experiences with POI vary and not all women feel this way, media and popular culture tell us over and over again that many women embrace menopause as an entry into a new (and sometimes even better) phase of life. Perhaps they are finding a new sense of self-assurance, feeling pride in grown children, and enjoying more free time. Who doesn't want all of that? But it is important to acknowledge that entry into menopause, at any age, can be a time of uncertainty and unwelcome change for some. Not all women find themselves with fewer responsibilities or greater personal wellbeing.

Women with POI experience many of the signs and symptoms of perimenopause and menopause, but none of the potential perks associated with this transition at midlife. Although most women experience some hard moments during the menopausal transition, POI brings with it additional or heightened uncertainties: negativity around loss of fertility, confused feelings about femininity, and overall shock at the early onset of this transition. Moreover, their doctors are not really sure what to think or do about it. Women are left wondering: "What the heck is going on with me? This is not supposed to be happening—not at this age, anyway! What am I to do regarding my future and how do I go on being a young woman, or engaging in friendships, dating, marriage, and motherhood?" Leah, age thirty-six, helps us understand these feelings:

After twenty years of regular monthly reminders that "I Am Woman," this absence of regularity is somewhat confusing. I'm thirty-six years old and part of what makes this tough is that a lot of people outside my support network have never heard about POI and don't always realize what I'm going through emotionally and physically. It feels like getting hit broadside by a speeding menopause bullet train to Hell, and you're up to your eyeballs with symptoms that make whacking yourself over the head with a two-by-four seem like a fun idea. Now what?

A Clinical Diagnosis

Women and their healthcare providers find that POI is often difficult to define, diagnose, and understand. The clinical progression of POI usually starts with sparse or infrequent (oligomenorrhea) or absent (amenorrhea) menstrual cycles for four months or more, in addition to high levels of follicle stimulating hormone (FSH) concentrations, which are considered well within the menopausal range (ACOG). In the majority of cases, the underlying cause for POI remains unknown even after thorough evaluations for medical causes. As a result, POI presents unique challenges for girls and women, their parents, and the clinicians who care for them. Although the diagnosis of POI is often significantly delayed due to the widely accepted assumption that irregular menses are common among adolescents and young women, early detection of this condition is crucial for the maintenance of overall health and wellbeing (especially for the prevention of more serious long-term conditions like bone loss, cardiovascular disease, and infertility) (ACOG; Pederson et al.).

What causes POI is poorly understood. In fact, in about 90 per cent of cases, the exact cause of POI remains a mystery (ACOG). However, some possible explanations have been identified. Some women are just born with fewer follicles in their ovaries, so eggs are depleted sooner. Genetic disorders such as fragile X syndrome and Turner syndrome can lead to POI (Nelson 610). Most women and girls with certain metabolic syndromes, such as galactosemia, also have POI (Nelson 611). Auto-immune diseases can sometimes damage the ovaries or the glands needed to make hormones to support the ovaries. About 20 per cent of women with POI also have an autoimmune disease, particularly thyroiditis (inflammation of the thyroid gland) or Addison's disease (which affects the adrenal glands) (Rebar 1360). Chemotherapy or radiation therapy can damage the genetic material in cells, including in the ovaries, causing them to stop working (Nelson 611). Pelvic surgery also may lead to the sudden impairment of ovarian function (Nelson 611). Environmental toxins—such as cigarette smoke, chemicals, and pesticides—have also been shown to affect ovarian function (De Vos et al. 913). All these contexts make individual POI experiences unique, complicating treatment. One woman's advice to others seeking healthcare highlights doctors' uncertainty about how to treat patients with POI:

> For those of you who have gone from doctor to doctor and taken one ineffective medication after another, I think the answer may be to learn as much as possible about your own body and how it works. I wasted so much time believing that the next doctor or naturopath was going to have the perfect answer. They all had a part of the truth, but I had to separate the wheat from the chaff. It's really too bad we don't get an owner's manual to tell us more, but we can learn by reading and discussion and sharing our success stories. (Jill, thirty-one)

Unfortunately, POI has no cure. Ovarian insufficiency cannot be reversed (American Academy of Pediatrics). Treatment options for POI have traditionally focused on hormonal therapy and fertility preservation. However, since most studies on menopause and related ovarian function recruit only older women as research participants, little data exist about the efficacy of POI treatments. Sparse information is available regarding the response of young women with POI to hormone therapy; this is true both in situations within which POI has explained causes (e.g., as the result of previous medical treatments or diagnoses) and unexplained causes (i.e., POI arises unexpectedly and without a specific cause). Even less is known about adolescents' responses to hormone therapy. Significant delays in diagnosis can exacerbate this knowledge deficit. Data are also scant regarding underlying genetic issues associated with POI (Chapman et al. 799). Perhaps more importantly, little research has focused on the emotional health of women experiencing POI across all age groups (Gordon et al. 511). Some women told us that patient-doctor interactions often made things worse, because doctors stick closely to blood test results and symptom checklists that do not always parallel the experiences of women with POI:

> I'm more than my ovaries, dammit. Every time I visit my doctor, he doesn't bother to look at me. He comes in the exam room, reviews my latest blood hormone levels, and tells me what medication changes he want to make. The last time I asked a question about a new symptom, he said ... "Now you know what women have been going through for thousands of years." What a slap in the face! (Tessa, twenty-nine)

Not Your Mother's Menopause

Menopause is defined as the permanent end of menstruation caused by the depletion of eggs (or more accurately the depletion of follicles—the fluid-filled cavities found in the wall of the ovary that contain the eggs or oocytes) (ACOG). How quickly this depletion occurs is up for debate, and it is impossible to predetermine each woman's perimeno-pausal trajectory. The average age of natural menopause is fifty-two years old but can vary depending on socioeconomic, lifestyle, and other health factors (Gold et al. 80). Women with POI are commonly compared to women who transition to menopause at midlife, without much thought given to differences in their experience. For instance, most adolescents and young women with POI do not exhibit permanent cessation of ovarian function and may experience intermittent and unpredictable ovarian activity for many years (Hubayter et al. 1770). Because POI, like menopause, is associated with low estrogen levels and other hormonal alterations, it can cause menopausal-type symptoms such as fatigue, hot flashes, altered sleep, dry-eye symptoms, and decreased libido (Gordon et al. 513). But since women typically go through menopause at midlife, healthcare providers are unaccustomed to explaining physical and laboratory findings in ways that reassure or make sense to young women with POI. Symptoms can start virtually overnight for some women, whereas for others, the changes are more gradual. Because many healthcare providers have never seen patients with this rare diagnosis, they fail to understand these signs and symptoms. This reality contributes to significant delays in diagnosis, treatment, and support, and leads to feelings of alienation and vulnerability for the young women experiencing them (Chapman et al.). As Christina, age nineteen, explains:

My mom joked once with my dad that if she didn't know better, she would have said that I was going through menopause at the time she was going through the same. However, Mom then shared the same joke with my doctor, who rather than trying to find out what on earth was going on with me referred me to a psychiatrist, as I was obviously seeking attention and mimicking my mother's symptoms. By this point, I was fourteen and heading into high school. All I wanted was to feel like a normal teenager talking about boys and enjoying music rather than discussing hot flashes.

Delayed diagnosis of POI is problematic especially for young women like Christina, since serious long-term medical consequences include increased risk for bone loss. Although bone loss is common among people over the age of fifty, women with POI may develop the condition at a much younger age. An adequate level of estrogen in the body is an important factor in promoting bone strength and preventing bone loss. Without appropriate estrogen levels, bone loss can lead to osteoporosis—a condition in which decreased bone density and strength results in significant risk of fracture. With POI, young women may fail to accrue their peak bone mass during a critical period for bone growth (Gordon et al. 262). Overall, adolescents and women with POI generally have lower bone mineral density (BMD) levels than healthy age-matched peers, and available evidence suggests the incidence of osteoporosis is much higher among women with POI compared to postmenopausal women (Popat et al. 2280). Liz, age twenty-three, makes it clear that bones are on the minds of doctors: "Bones, bones, bones. I would be happy if my doctor never mentioned the word again. It is the bone concern that keeps me awake at night wondering what is the best thing to do to protect my bones? I've seen what osteoporosis can do, and it scares me. I don't want to be the lady who is all hunched over because I was not willing to talk to my doctor, especially at my age."

Although some symptoms of POI and age-appropriate menopause can be similar, such as the loss of bone density, there is nothing normal or natural about POI. It is completely unexpected, often embarrassing and stigmatizing, and definitely not part of the natural aging process experienced by older women. Thinking about POI as just early menopause is not always helpful in understanding what girls and young women go through. Whereas many middle-aged women learn about menopause from their mothers, older relatives, or friends, there is no comparable opportunity for women with POI. Most do not know anyone else with the condition; they have no one to go to for sage advice, which leads to feelings of isolation and hesitancy to disclose or talk about one's condition. Marybeth, age twenty-six, discusses the importance of gaining more information and support from the beginning in order to "come to ... peace" with a POI diagnosis:

> The best decision I've made so far about POI is this: I made sure I educated myself about POI. I talked about it with people. When I first found out, I felt very alone. I didn't know that there were other people out there in the same situation. I've also come to some sort of peace with this. It has taken me a long time. I allow myself to cry about it when I feel down about it, but I also reach out when I need help. The good thing is, I know I'm not alone.

Although natural menopause in a middle-aged woman is not always celebrated, it is a predictable milestone within the life course of adulthood. Camaraderie between middle-aged women facing and managing the symptomatic consequences of perimenopause can make the discomforts easier to endure. Women with POI miss out on this experience. Dealing with a POI diagnosis can be further complicated for adolescents and young women because parents, perhaps especially mothers, may be coming to terms with the diagnosis at the same time. It can be heartbreaking for a mother to watch her young daughter face a diagnosis with implications beyond her understanding. Yet a mother's attitude plays a vital role in how a young woman processes POI (Sterling and Best-Boss 190). Sometimes a mother's own grief may overshadow her daughter's feelings. This can be true for several reasons. POI might be genetically based, so a mother may feel guilt for passing along faulty genes. She may mourn the loss of potential grandchildren or worry about long-term complications to her daughter's health. Some mothers withdraw, perhaps overwhelmed by the uncertainties that lie ahead for their daughters. Living with POI will reveal further layers of vulnerability over the next several decades. When mothers cannot cope effectively with the implications of this condition, their daughters are left feeling more isolated. Girls and young women with POI need to see themselves reflected in others' eyes, especially the eyes of their mothers, as being whole, lovable, healthy, young women:

I was fourteen years old. And short. And flat chested. It did not bother me until my younger sister started getting a regular period and got taller than I was. She tried to hide it, but it seemed so unfair that she was growing and changing, and I had just stopped. I started stuffing my bras with tissues to make myself bigger and lying about my period, but I felt like a freak. The first doctor that my mother took me to said that I was just a "late bloomer" and did everything but pat me on my head and send us away. Luckily, my mom did not give up and kept trying until she found a doctor who would listen and actually do some tests. While we were glad to have some answers, we ended up with a lot more questions. Going through menopause in high school was not easy. I tried to be a regular teenager, but I began having hot flashes, nightly sweats, mood swings, and sleepless nights too. At least, we now know what we are up against. (Susanna, age eighteen)

The emotional adjustments associated with POI also make POI distinct from normal experiences of perimenopause and menopause. Every aspect of a woman's life is affected by a POI diagnosis. Not understanding what is wrong, feeling a lack of control over symptoms, and not knowing what the future holds can be frightening. Initially, she may doubt her femininity or womanhood and feel as if she is watching her own body dissolve. Long-held beliefs and views about the world and reality might be called into question. According to interviews, some women talk of a "loss of womanhood" and the "loss of dreams" in their twenties and thirties, with fifty to sixty years left in their lives to live (Sterling and Best-Boss 157), which suggests they are not always emotionally prepared to face their diagnosis. Adolescent girls and young women with POI feel estranged; they know that their ovaries are malfunctioning and fear future complications. Sudden news of infertility can cause psychological distress and anxiety, and impair self-esteem. The most common words women use to describe their emotional state after being diagnosed with POI are "devastated," "shocked," and "confused" (Groff et al. 1738). Many women we interviewed talked about reimagining their futures:

I've finally discovered there is too little time to punish oneself for conditions one cannot control. I've chosen to lead a life in which I'm active in the things I can control as well as accepting the

things I cannot. I cannot control my primary ovarian insufficiency, but I can control my attitude towards it. I hope to share
this attitude with others in the hope that they, too, one day will
accept themselves for who they are and not for the POI they
carry. POI is a part of my life, but is it not my life. (Carly, age
thirty-two)

Another spoke to the emotional adjustment women diagnosed with
POI must experience:

The best advice anyone gave me: Don't make any rash decisions.
Upon learning your diagnosis, you will probably go through a
series of emotions, including denial, devastation, regret, anger,
and/or depression. It takes time before your body and mind have
time to adjust. Take your time, before you make any major
decisions about what you want to do with your life, particularly
concerning family building. (Jill, age twenty-seven)

For all of these reasons, POI is not your mother's menopause. Increasing awareness about this condition, and its management, will lead to
advances in both emotional and physical care. Access to short-term
resources, such as referrals to appropriate counselling services, along
with long-term follow-up care, is critically important to helping young
women and their families navigate the challenges of living with POI.

Family Planning after POI Diagnosis

We have all heard about the proverbial biological clock and the
reproductive transitions women are supposed to encounter at different
life stages. You get your first period at twelve or fourteen and suddenly
become a fertile woman. You spend your young adulthood trying to
prevent pregnancy. At some point, you throw away your birth control
to have a baby. Motherhood and, if you're lucky, grandmotherhood
follow. You transition to menopause, settle into retirement, and perhaps
take up new hobbies or pursue fresh adventures with your newfound
freedom. Isn't this what every happy, healthy woman should aspire to?
It certainly is not the pathway that unfurls for women with POI.

Today, many women's lives are too complicated to be tied up into neat
little boxes. Some women seek partners; others do not. Some desire

children, whereas others choose to remain childfree. Others attempt to have biological children and find out that they cannot conceive. Our lives are affected by a myriad of factors—such as education, employment, finances, relationships, and overall health—and do not follow a pre-scribed path to the same milestones. This is especially true for women with POI, whose choices are even more limited:

> I know it's tough—any and all of us who have dealt with this whole POI thing has grappled with the "Am I still sexy? Am I still a woman? Am I still what I thought I was?" stuff. And from one who has been there and come out on the other end, all I want to share with you is that you are so much more than ovaries or ability to reproduce or whatever. I know, I know…it is easy for me to say since I have gotten past it, but it's true. (Lisa, age forty)

Some women we interviewed were cognizant of their biological clocks. As much as we might like to deny it, the biological clock in many ways is still alive and ticking. Our reproductive organs and abilities are on a deadline heavily influenced by the passage of time. Theoretically we start our periods at a certain time, attempt to become pregnant at a certain time, and, at a certain time in midlife, cease being able to reproduce. Unfortunately, some of us have little warning or control over when or if these things will happen. Each of us is influenced by different factors, many of which are out of our control. In the end, we may have no idea how our biological clocks will wind down, as mentioned by Veronica, age twenty-six: "One doctor said to me that there are two areas of the human body that we don't yet fully understand. One of these is the brain. The other, of course, is women's hormonal system."

Realizing POI has affected your fertility and that having a child may not be as easy as one hoped can be traumatic. Because women with POI may occasionally ovulate, it is possible to become pregnant without the assistance of fertility treatments. However, only about 5 to 10 per cent of women with POI do become pregnant spontaneously (Bidet et al. 2864), and this is usually just a matter of luck. Most women with POI must seek out a fertility specialist if they want to become pregnant. Because women with POI do not produce many eggs, using an egg donor is often recommended for women who desire to become pregnant. Other options for family building include surrogacy, embryo donation, and adoption (Egbe et al.). But fertility treatments are expensive, emotionally and physically exhausting, and inaccessible for some due to the limited availability of specialists. As POI gets more attention, researchers are now looking at possible ways to reverse POI by addressing hormone levels to maximize ovarian reserve or preserve fertility (Rafique et al. 584). For now, women like Amber, age thirty-seven, are dealing with the possibility they cannot have children who are biologically related to them:

> My experience with POI started when I was thirty-three, when my fiancé and I decided we wanted to have a baby. Within two months of that decision, and up until then, my periods has [sic] always been what I thought was normal. I started skipping periods. At first, I thought it might be stress of working on having a baby, as I've always been a high-stress individual—so I figured I would focus on relaxing to see if that would change things. After a few months, I went to my doctor. My doctor is a great guy; however, when it came to telling me that I had POI, I actually read his diagnosis on the referral sheet to the fertility doctor—he never said a word. The sheet read that I should have an ultrasound to look at my ovaries due to ovarian FAILURE. I sat for a good hour in the parking lot and cried. I was unaware of ovaries failing—I had in my head that everyone my age could have a baby except for a very small amount of women. I found that to be the total opposite. I had to deal with the fact that there wouldn't be any babies naturally, and that was very hard. I still believe we will have little ones in our lives. I just do not know how that will happen yet.

Losing the possibility of biological motherhood may be heartbreaking for women like Amber. However, other women in our study remained ambivalent, making comments like "I wasn't sure if I even wanted children" and "I didn't know if I wanted more children." The biggest frustration for most women we interviewed was having their choice for biological motherhood taken away. But the major emotional impacts of the diagnosis for most young women are shock at the news of loss of normal fertility and grief over the loss of future dreams and aspirations. Biological motherhood, whether longed for or not, might not be possible—at least not easily. Feelings of shame and embarrassment can compound the emotional impact:

I never really told any of my friends [about my POI and its impact on fertility]. I told one who did not know what to say or do, and the conversation was dropped, so I decided it was best not to bother. If I'm completely honest about it, I did and still do feel almost ashamed about it, even though I know I haven't done anything wrong. It is still something I feel embarrassed about and have a hard time talking about. (Karen, age thirty)

POI also can have a significant impact on relationships, current and future, partly because it can be difficult to conceptualize a life without motherhood and family. Women with partners might need to redefine plans, goals, expectations, and dreams. Women not yet in committed relationships have another challenge: How do you tell a new partner you are going through menopause at age twenty and might not be able to have children? In addition, friends and family may withdraw because they do not know how to respond or assume saying nothing is better than saying the wrong thing. A supportive primary relationship can make a big difference:

Many people suspect my condition, but because POI is a closed issue, they don't like to ask. And I don't want to rush in and confide in others. If my work colleagues knew I was menopausal and infertile, then they would feel uncomfortable, especially talking about their children. My husband has been a great support and accompanied me on my journey. In fact, if it hadn't been for him, I know I would have crumbled a long time ago. (Sherri, thirty-three)

Unfortunately, our interviews made clear that the kind of support Sherri receives from her husband is not widespread.

The Menstrual Cycle as a Vital Sign

Perhaps most importantly, the menstrual cycle is about more than fertility and reproduction. In 2006, the American Academy of Pediatrics and the American College of Obstetricians and Gynecologists published a clinical report on menstruation in girls and adolescents that stated in the abstract: "Using the menstrual cycle as an additional vital sign adds a powerful tool to the assessment of normal development and the exclusion of pathological conditions" (AAP and ACOG). As

POI experts know, irregular menstrual cycles among adolescents and young women can be a significant indicator of endocrine problems or other serious health issues (Pederson). It is important to find the cause of irregular or absent menstrual cycles. Taking a wait-and-see attitude or, worse yet, masking conditions with inappropriately prescribed hormonal birth control or other medications without a complete and accurate diagnosis can have potentially debilitating or even life-threatening effects. In addition to POI, causes of irregular or absent menstrual cycles among young women and adolescents may include eating disorders and exercise-induced amenorrhea as well as conditions like a pituitary tumour (AAP and ACOG). Currently, too many women and their healthcare providers believe that regarding menstrual cycles, it is fine not to have menstrual periods. But menstrual irregularity can have significant adverse consequences over the long term, particularly related to bone loss. Because few talk openly about menstruation, young women and their healthcare providers are often unsure about what represents normal menstrual patterns and are often unclear about normal ranges for cycle length, amount, and duration of flow. Lack of knowledge around menstruation is due largely to ignorance and shame about the menstrual cycle (Johnston-Robledo et al. 25). Like other vital signs for detecting health issues—pulse rate, body temperature, blood pressure, and respiratory rate—the menstrual cycle is a valuable tool for assessing women's overall health and wellbeing that should not be ignored. Not all doctors understand this, as illustrated by one woman's long road to diagnosis:

> For years, I knew something just wasn't right. I explained my missing periods and other symptoms to doctor after doctor. Everyone just dismissed it and said we would "deal" with it once I wanted to have a baby. One even told me that I was lucky not to have a period every month. After about ten years, I finally got a diagnosis of POI and then things started making sense. I hope that this delay won't impact my health in the long term, after all both my mom and grandmother had osteoporosis. I can't tell you how much I wish I had found out sooner. I wouldn't have wondered and worried so much about my health. I'm happy to report that I found a great doctor that takes me seriously and understands that periods are more than just for getting pregnant. (Shayna, age thirty-seven)

Shayna's story tells us how important it is for doctors to take menstrual cycle problems seriously. Early diagnosis of POI is a first step to improving care and support for adolescents and women with this condition.

An Integrative Approach to POI

POI is a serious chronic condition, lasting decades, with far-reaching health implications. Early diagnosis, effective POI-specific treatments, and a broad range of family-building options will help women with POI live long, healthy, happy lives. Communities of support also are needed to help lessen the emotional and psychological impacts many adolescents and young women experience. Clinicians need to commit to treating the whole person throughout her lifetime, not just during the initial POI diagnosis. All this considered, we believe that a multi-disciplinary, collaborative, and integrative approach to POI is required to promote the overall health and wellbeing for women across all life stages. With advancing knowledge and integrated resources, young women will not have to make their own way as Elaine, age fifty, once did:

At age fifty, it feels odd to be considered a long-term survivor of POI. But that is indeed what I am. To have been diagnosed at age twenty-nine, I've had twenty years of trial and error and deep reflection to discover what works best for me. But, boy, did I feel isolated twenty plus years ago when the doctor first told me of my diagnosis and that there was "nobody" to whom I could talk to who also had POI because it was "extremely rare." Today, I am more energetic, happier, and more positive than ever before.

An integrative approach to POI should develop broader definitions of perimenopause and menopause that extend the boundaries of menopause discourse to include the voices of younger women. Although all menopausal women share some similar experiences, women under the age of forty represent a distinct group with different needs and additional complicated issues. We also need to develop multidisciplinary resources to address the overlapping physical, emotional, and social changes patients experience. Young women need more detailed information about how to live well throughout a lifetime with early menopause, particularly as things change across the life course (Rafique 567; Sterling 235).

Most importantly, we should provide opportunities for women living with POI to share their unique perspectives and personal stories. POI is much more than a physical experience or clinical diagnosis; it hits women at their very core, eliciting powerful feelings of embarrassment, isolation, and stigma. For researchers and all care providers to better understand the vast impact of POI, descriptions of women's lived experiences need to accompany scientific information about the condition, which will normalize and provide context to women's experiences, as we have done here. Women with POI need no longer be passive bystanders. Instead, they can voice their concerns and accomplishments, make informed decisions, and seek out advice, support, and treatment that will make them stronger and healthier:

> My diagnosis was unexpected and unwelcome. Nevertheless, my POI had a strange, uplifting effect on my life. I now recognize the importance of life and what a gift it truly is. Every day that goes by, I'm thankful for being alive. Don't get me wrong, like probably all women with POI, every day that goes by, I continue to wish that my diagnosis could be reversed. Yes, I still long and wish for my fertility back. Yes, I worry about my hormone levels, my bone loss, my early aging, and all the other things that come along with POI. But now, I see every day as a learning day. I continually search for new ways to deal with POI, and I will continue to work on my treatment regimen (which needs to be routinely updated and refined). POI is not something that I can change or cure, so I'm learning to live with it the best possible way. (Kaye, age thirty-seven)

Not all paths to menopause are straightforward, predictable, or even welcomed. Although all women experience decline in ovarian function and menstrual cycle disruptions over time, for adolescents and young women with POI, these changes come too soon. As this chapter makes clear, they face additional challenges beyond those of women who go through the menopausal transition at midlife. An integrative approach to POI that places women at the centre is key to addressing all aspects of their intertwined emotional and physical health. All women deserve the best possible health at every age and phase of life.

Works Cited

American Academy of Pediatrics (AAP), Committee on Adolescence and the American College of Obstetricians and Gynecologists (ACOG), and the Committee on Adolescent Health Care. "Menstruation in Girls and Adolescents: Using the Menstrual Cycle as a Vital Sign." *Pediatrics* vol. 118, no. 5, 2006, pediatrics.aappublications.org/content/118/5/2245.short. Accessed 1 Oct. 2017.

American College of Obstetricians and Gynecologists (ACOG) and the Committee on Adolescent Health Care. "Committee Opinion: Primary Ovarian Insufficiency in Adolescents and Young Women." *ACOG*, 2014, www.acog.org/Resources-And-Publications/Committee-Opinions/Committee-on-Adolescent-Health-Care/Primary-Ovarian-Insufficiency-in-Adolescents-and-Young-Women. Accessed 1 Oct. 2017.

Bidet, Maud, et al. "Resumption of Ovarian Function and Pregnancies in 358 Patients with Premature Ovarian Failure." *Journal of Clinical Endocrinology & Metabolism*, vol. 96, no. 1, 2011, pp. 3864-72.

Chapman, Chevy, Lynsey Cree, and Andrew N. Shelling. "The Genetics of Premature Ovarian Failure: Current Perspectives". *International Journal of Women's Health*, vol. 7, 2015, pp. 799-810.

Covington, Sharon, et al.. "A Family Systems Approach to Primary Ovarian Insufficiency." *Journal of Pediatric and Adolescent Gynecology*, vol. 24, no. 3, 2011, pp. 137-41.

De Vos, Michel, Paul Devroey, and Bart Fauser. "Primary Ovarian Insufficiency." *Lancet,* vol. 376, no. 9744, 2010, pp. 911-21.

Egbe, Thomas Obinchemti, et al. "Successful Pregnancy with Donor Eggs In-Vitro Fertilization after Premature Ovarian Insufficiency in a Tertiary Hospital in a Low Income Setting: A Case Report." *Fertility Research & Practice*, vol. 2, no. 12, 2016, fertilityresearchandpractice.biomedcentral.com/articles/10.1186/s40738-016-0028-3. Accessed 1 Oct. 2017.

Gold, Ellen, et al. "Factors Related to Age at Natural Menopause: Longitudinal Analyses from SWAN." *American Journal of Epidemiology,* vol. 178, no. 1, 2013, pp. 70-83.

Gordon, Catherine, B. S. Zemel, and T. A. Wren. "The Determinants of Peak Bone Mass." *Journal of Pediatrics,* vol. 180, 2017, pp. 261-69.

Gordon, Catherine, Tsuzuki Kanaoka, and Lawrence Nelson. "Update on Primary Ovarian Insufficiency in Adolescents." *Current Opinions in Pediatrics,* vol. 26, no. 4, 2015, pp. 511-19.

Groff, Alison, et al. "Assessing the Emotional Needs of Women with Spontaneous Premature Ovarian Failure." *Fertility and Sterility,* vol. 83, no. 6, 2005, pp. 1734-41.

Hubayter, Ziad, et al. "A Prospective Evaluation of Antral Follicle Function in Women with 46, XX Spontaneous Primary Ovarian Insufficiency." *Fertility and Sterility,* vol. 94, no. 5, 2010, pp. 1769-74.

Johnston-Robledo, Ingrid, et al "Reproductive Shame: Self-Objectification and Young Women's Attitudes Toward Their Reproductive Functioning." *Women & Health,* vol. 46, no. 1, 2007, pp. 25-39.

Nelson, Lawrence. "Primary Ovarian Insufficiency." *New England Journal of Medicine,* vol. 360, no. 6, 2009, pp. 606-14.

Pederson, Julia, et al. "Primary Ovarian Insufficiency in Adolescents: A Case Series." *International Journal of Endocrinology,* vol. 13, 2015, ijpeonline.biomedcentral.com/articles/10.1186/s13633-015-0009 -z. Accessed 1 Oct. 2017.

Popat, Vaishali, et al. "Bone Mineral Density in Estrogen-Deficient Young Women." *Journal of Clinical Endocrinology Metabolism,* vol. 94, no. 7, 2009, pp. 2277-83.

Rafique, Saima, Evelina W. Sterling, and Lawrence M. Nelson. "A New Approach to Primary Ovarian Insufficiency." *Obstet Gynecol Clin North Am,* vol. 39, no. 4, 2012, pp. 567-86.

Rebar, Robert. "Premature Ovarian Failure." *Obstetrics and Gynecology,* vol. 113, no. 6, 2009, pp. 1355-63.

Sterling, Evelina, and Angie Best-Boss. *Before Your Time: The Early Menopause Survival Guide."* Simon & Schuster, 2010.

Welt, Corrine. "Primary Ovarian Insufficiency: A More Accurate Term for Premature Ovarian Failure." *Clinical Endocrinology,* vol. 68, no. 4, 2008, pp. 499-509.

Chapter 7

Shadow Story

Yolanda Kauffman

D arkness descended on my life after learning that my body
(without consulting with my heart, mind, and soul) had started
the journey of early menopause at the age of thirty-two. Since
that time, I have put much effort into transforming a devastating and
painful thirteen-year event into a mystical and powerful experience
from which I continue to grow and learn.

Making photographs has been a creative outlet and meditative
practice for me since I was young. The use of shadows to tell my story
provides depth, symbolism, and expanded awareness that words cannot
express. Facing into my shadows is how I found my creative womb. By
shining the light of awareness on the dark years of my soul, I awaken.

May my story invite you to an awakening as you consciously
engage your menopause journey.
May it open you into the mystery and power of menopause.
May you find, trust and give voice to the wisdom that emerges
from menopause.
May you revel in the alchemy of menopause.
May you allow your authentic being to rise from menopause.
May you welcome others to join in this process of transformation.
May it be so.

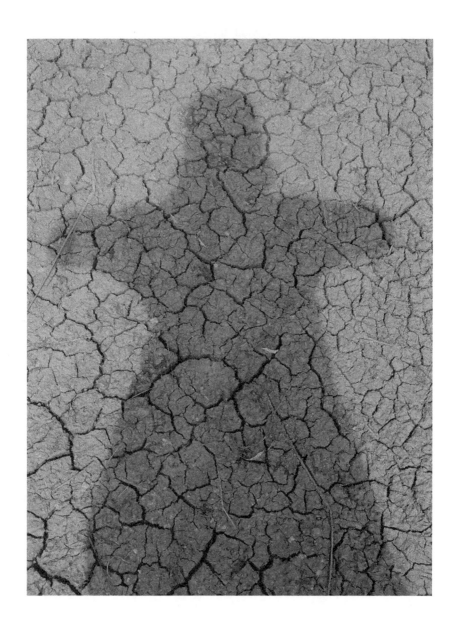

Becoming Conscious

Becoming conscious
of

F	E	A	R
e	x	l	e
e	t	t	a
l	r	e	l
i	e	r	i
n	m	e	t
g	e	d	y

Experiencing an internal, invisible, shape-shifting metamorphosis,
that was unacknowledged and denied,
emotional survival was the root of my existence.
Deep grief.
Shattered dreams.
Broken.
Alone.

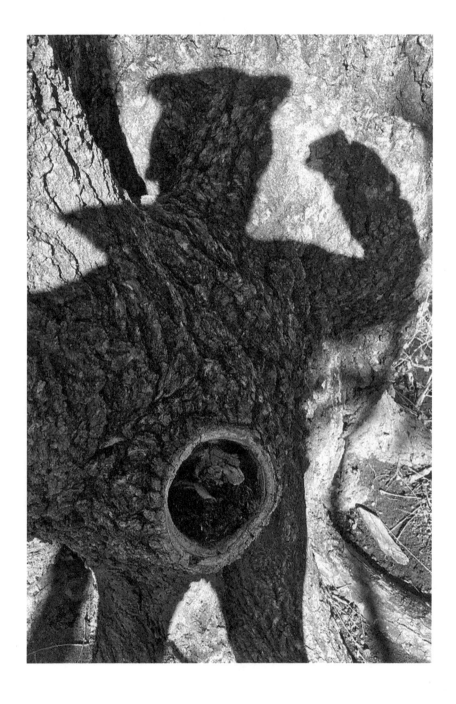

Moontime Explosion

Fertile tides recede
creativity abounds.
Synapses dissolve
energy ignites.
Fire in the womb!
Power to the pussy!
Power to the pause!
Power to the portal!
As the waves crest
so shall I rise.

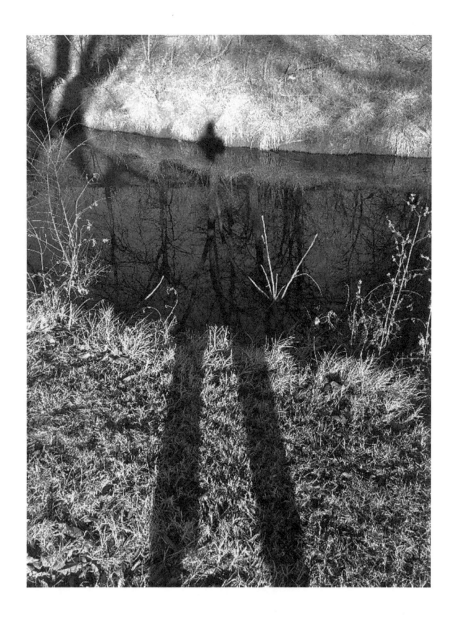

Witnessing

With mind, body, and soul wide open
I listen.
Freeing myself
from emotional toxicity.
Willing negatives into positives.
Being mindful of my propensity to judge.

Confidence builds,
identity blossoms.
I
see.

Witnessing.
I claim my power.
Vibrations ripple.
Juices flow.
I am cleansed,
as deep passion burns.

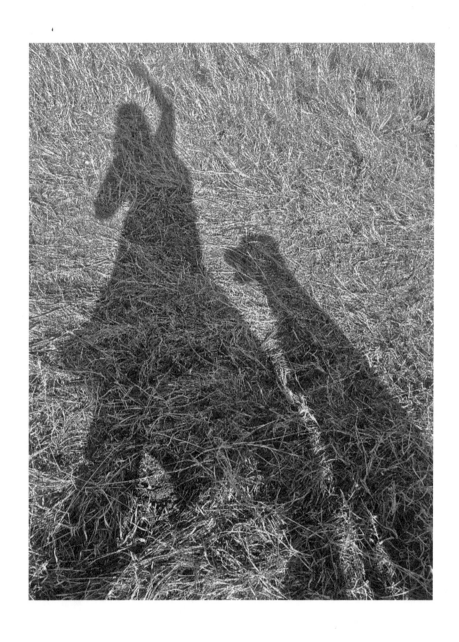

Dance of Love

Trusting myself
to ride
the current of transformation.
Letting go of the past,
spinning into the unknown.
Binding my heart to this new tide.
Never alone.
Flying free.

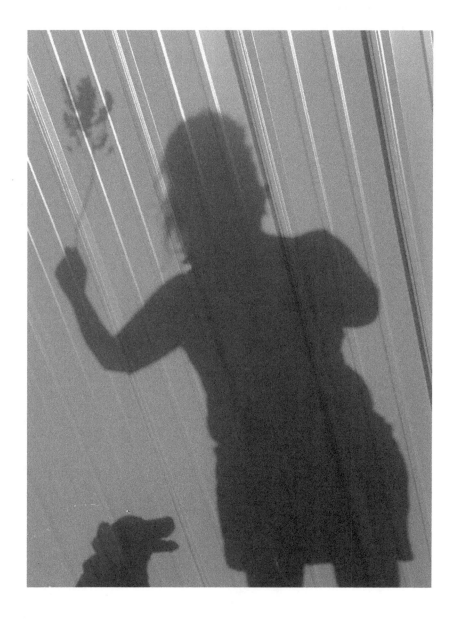

Writing on the Wall

i

have a voice

i

am powerful

i

claim my authority

i

am fluent in the energies of my body

i

am open

i

explore

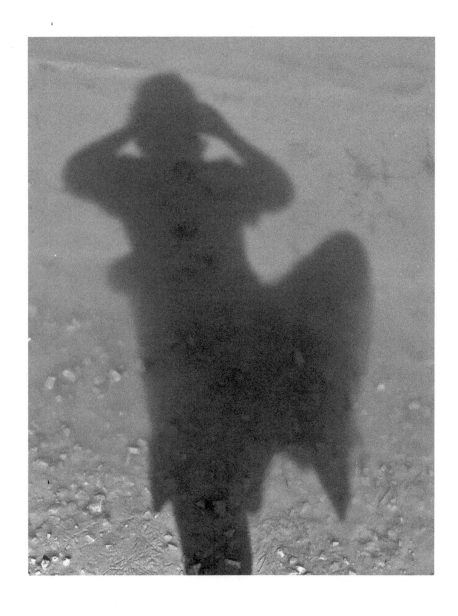

Clear Sight

Delving into my shadows,
awareness expands.

Connecting to my inner knowledge,
insight arises.

Following my breath,
visions are found.

Smelling the muskiness of truth,
illumination bubbles.

Tasting the nectar of life,
energy permeates.

There is no edge to this awareness.

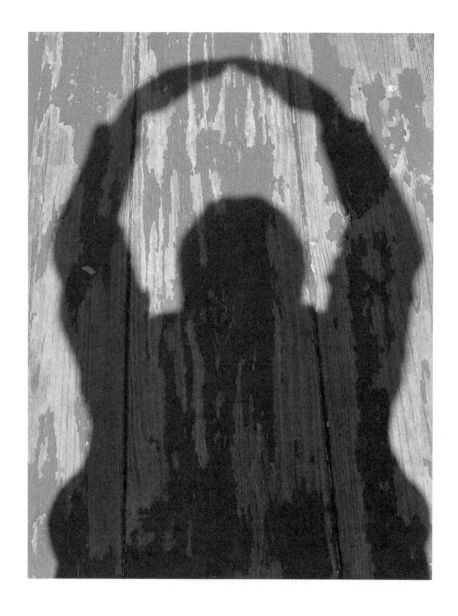

The Intention of Crones

we
consciously circle

to
revolutionize

our
oneness

holding
stories

embodying
sanctity.

Chapter 8

Just before Menopause

Donna J. Gelagotis Lee

Forty-one

Too young for menopause, the doctor says
as I look at a picture of his wife, almost
my age, and wonder what he'll be telling her
if she wakes up in a sweat one night

and begins not to be able to sleep, her body,
which she had always known, beginning to behave
erratically. I understand my own body, I think, and
I will never be back to this

fine doctor. I will never come back,
I'm thinking, will never see these
efficient office workers, this cozy waiting
room, these large doors to the outside.

Forty-two

Six months of reading and apprehending.
Doctor two: It could be menopause,
though you're young. I *knew*... Didn't
know why I needed her to say it.

No medication for this.
Drenching my nightgown one, two times
a night. If I don't get relief now,
will I ever be able to? I don't

want to conceive, only the option to.
Does the ability make one feel
vital, desirable? What
is the power of sex?

Forty-three

Books appear on perimenopause. At least
I'm "current." *Soy* becomes a catchword.
I try soy pills, black cohosh. I try
exercise. I try OTC meds to sleep.

I sleep with an extra nightgown
under my pillow. I can almost
change nightgowns in my sleep. My friends
are getting pregnant.

My friends are not getting hot
flashes, are not having trouble sleeping,
are not thinking about getting old
and being childless forever.

Forty-four

The internet gives me lots of hits—
blood clots?—no, not pulmonary—

menarche?—no, not girls starting—
fibroids?—no, not heavy bleeding—

clots?—light, prolonged bleeding—
cancer?—God, hope not, no—

menopause? I hit an electronic mailing list
and that's where the symptoms make

sense—described by other women—
why didn't someone tell us?

Forty-five

I see the image of my mother
in the mirror as I pass.
I am only forty-five, but feel more
like eighteen inside.

What part of the brain
rehearses youth? I can't believe
the stray moment kicking in the corner.
Why is the present always the present

while time ages us slowly, almost
imperceptibly. I pass by the mirror,
time lurking. Yet the mirror sees
no ghosts.

Forty-six

Is it a dream, melatonin
inspired? Or a night sweat
of menopause? The double
hour, an alarm within,
as if something should
happen...

Shallow nightmare, go!
I am oddly willing to concede.
Yet my body intervenes,
logging sleep. Thank
goodness, it's smarter
than me.

Forty-seven

Perimenopause—
not quite feeling
my old self.

Forty-eight

Give me some HRT with no
increased risk of stroke,

VTE, or cancer. Give me
my health, not simply my

youth. I fear death
is lassoing in. Doctor, give me

more than fifteen minutes.
I'm too tired to come back four more

times. And I'll forget what I wanted
to say.

Forty-nine

The doctor tries to readjust,
            substituting feeling
lousy with feeling
            different.

But *she's* years shy
            of menopause. How
could she conceive of
            slowing down, re-

versing, the body in midlife
            adolescence? You'd like
her to admit, *Yes, it can be like PMS
            all of the time,*

but worse—

Fifty

—breakouts
        in places you've never had them—
and just when lack of sleep
        was your chief complaint,

move over—and not to your partner's
        side of the bed—he's
staying clear of this— hot/cold—
        temperature

as uncertain as menstruation—
        someone should tell you
how the skin thins,
        how the muscle

you once simply flexed
        now requires
weight training to maintain
        strength—

how the body makes decisions,
        the body that houses you,
ageless and beautiful
        as you are.

Chapter 9

Patches Not Pads: An Intersex Experience with Postsurgical (Pseudo) Menopause

Georgiann Davis and Koyel Khan

M enopause often marks a transition in a woman's life, as it did for me, Georgiann. Only I was a teenager when doctors surgically shaped my body leaving me in what they labelled "postsurgical menopause." I was born intersex, but like other intersex people, I was not told the truth when I was diagnosed (e.g., Davis; Holmes; Karkazis; Preves). Instead, I was told I had underdeveloped malignant ovaries that needed to be removed. I have a vagina, but internally instead of XX chromosomes, ovaries, fallopian tubes, and a uterus, I have XY chromosomes and testes—that is until doctors surgically removed them because a girl is not supposed to have them. I weave my personal experience with intersex with a qualitative sociological analysis of how intersex is experienced and contested in contemporary American society in my book *Contesting Intersex: The Dubious Diagnosis* (Davis). In this chapter, sociologist Koyel Khan and I collaborate to draw on the intersex experience, specifically my experience, to offer a blended autoethnographic and life history account that exemplifies how, like menstruation (Hasson), menopause is also socially constructed.

Sociologist Sara Crawley defines autoethnography "as a kind of self-interview, which is not a defined method with specific parameters but rather a balancing act between modernist empirical science, postmodern deconstructions of science and subjectivity, and the activist pursuit of recording marginalized ideas and voices" (144). Psychologist John Dollard defines life history as the study of growth in one's life in order to make theoretical sense of their experiences. Although we depart from traditional autoethnography to co-author this chapter together, we do so under a mutual understanding and hope that a collaborative approach will enhance this hybrid autoethnographic and life history discussion of menopause as a socially constructed phenomenon.

When we say menopause is socially constructed, we are not denying that many females will experience a time in their life when their periods end, nor are we suggesting that peri- or postmenopausal experiences, such as hot flashes, are fictions of one's imagination (see Obermeyer). As critical feminists, we do not feel it is our place to challenge biological processes or question lived experiences. Rather, building on work that sees menopause in relation to medicalization processes (see Bell, "Sociological Perspectives on the Medicalization of Menopause") and its feminist challenges (Leng), we rely on an intersex experience to show how doctors draw on and reconstruct their definition of menopause to control who can experience menopause. This power over menopause allows doctors who treat intersex people to leverage their authority over biological processes while simultaneously minimizing how they are violating human rights when they perform medically unnecessary and irreversible interventions on intersex people's bodies.

We begin our discussion with a brief overview of intersex, including its changing nomenclature, to make the case that it is not unusual for doctors to reframe diagnoses, in this case menopause, to fit a narrative they are constructing. We then turn to a discussion of how doctors have historically, and horrifically, treated intersex people. Georgiann's experience is just one example of how doctors lie to intersex people about their diagnosis out of fear that knowing the truth would disrupt the development of an intersex person's gender identity. Next, we describe what it was like for Georgiann to navigate menopause without ever experiencing a period. More specifically, we explain how many intersex people, like Georgiann, are strongly compelled by their doctors to purchase expensive hormone replacement therapy (HRT) patches not covered by health insurance rather than pads from the feminine products aisle of their local grocery store. Many intersex people also face difficulty in finding the right hormonal balance for their body, leaving a number of intersex people, Georgiann included, altogether rejecting HRT. We conclude that the intersex experience highlighted here is a prime example of how menopause is a socially constructed phenomenon. Many intersex women never experience periods, yet as part of the powerful medical institution, doctors wrongly tell intersex people that they are in postsurgical menopause.

Understanding Intersex

All fetuses begin gestational development as intersex, meaning they are not neatly male or female. If a given fetus has XY chromosomes, it will be inundated with a substantial amount of androgens that will, in the average circumstance, shape the body's internal and external genitalia to resemble a male body with external testes and a penis. However, in some instances, a fetus with XY chromosomes is insensitive to androgens, resulting in a body with external genitalia that is not typically male. These folks are born with an intersex trait known as androgen insensitivity syndrome, or AIS for short. Depending upon the level of insensitivity to androgens, some people with XY chromosomes will be born with externally "ambiguous" genitalia. In such situations, it is likely they will be diagnosed with partial androgen insensitivity syndrome (PAIS). As the diagnostic terminology suggests, the body only partially responds to androgens. Those whose body is completely insensitive to androgens, like Georgiann, are typically born with what appears to be a vagina, but inside, instead of ovaries, a uterus, and fallopian tubes, they will have testes. These folks are said to have complete androgen insensitivity syndrome (CAIS). In this later case, the intersex trait often goes undi-agnosed until the absence of menstruation prompts further examination. The Intersex Society of North America has identified nearly twenty different intersex traits.[1]

Unfortunately, we do not have any reliable estimates of intersex in the population. However, attempts at estimating intersex have been made with a commonly cited statistic suggesting that on average, 2 per cent of live births are intersex (making it as common as being born with red hair), with roughly 0.1 to 0.2 per cent of live births resulting in "ambiguous" genitalia (Blackless et al.). Although the frequency of intersex in the population is understudied and unreliable, we do know that intersex is common enough that every single person on this planet has met someone who has been intersex—whether or not that intersex person was aware of their difference and felt comfortable disclosing their intersex status is, of course, a different story.

We also know that intersex has been documented in medical literature dating as far back as the eighteenth century (Warren). Intersex was historically referred to as hermaphroditism (Kessler, *Lessons from the Intersexed*), but that term is considered derogatory to some, though not all, intersex people today (Davis). Eventually, the term "intersex" took the place of "hermaphrodite" language in both medical and sociocultural scholarship (see, for example, Committee on Genetics; Dreger; Preves). As described in *Contesting Intersex* (Davis), 1990s intersex activism was successfully challenging medical authority over intersex. Intersex activists were appearing across media platforms to raise intersex visibility and share just how horrifically doctors were treating intersex people. With these challenges popping up across venues, medical authority over intersex was in jeopardy. The only way doctors could reassert their authority and reclaim jurisdiction over the intersex body was to reinvent the diagnosis, which the medical profession did in 2006 did by renaming intersex a disorder of sex development (Lee et al.). Doctors no longer fix intersex traits. They now treat disorders of sex development. This renaming of intersex throughout history is strong evidence that diagnoses are often reinvented, or reframed, to fit a particular narrative that maintains medical authority (Davis). And, as we shall show later in this chapter, doctors similarly reinvent the menopause narrative whenever they believe it necessary in order to explain the postsurgical lives of intersex people and to justify the medically unnecessary and irreversible interventions they have performed on intersex bodies.

Medical Lies

Doctors typically diagnose intersex at birth in the case of "ambiguous" genitalia or during adolescence when they search for an explanation of amenorrhea, the medical term for the absence of menstruation. Georgiann was diagnosed in the early 1990s when she was about thirteen years old. She was experiencing abdominal pain. Her mother initially thought Georgiann was getting her period, but then after her mother realized that was not what was happening, she took her to an urgent care centre for further examination. After a physical examination supplemented with medical imaging tests, it was quickly determined that Georgiann's abdominal pain was muscle related from running around outside. However, in the process of discovering nothing was wrong with Georgiann, the doctors uncovered that she was born without a uterus, fallopian tubes, and ovaries. Blood tests revealed that she had XY chromosomes, which confirmed their suspicion that she was intersex.

Georgiann clearly remembers the moment of final diagnosis. Her mother was hysterical, and Georgiann found herself comforting her mother at the urgent care centre At the time of the diagnosis, doctors lied to Georgiann as they did, and do, with so many other intersex people (Davis; Holmes; Karkazis; Preves; Davis and Feder). They told Georgiann that she would never be able to have children and that she had early onset ovarian cancer. The doctors assured Georgiann she would not die from the cancer, so she did not understand why her mother was so upset. Of course, she was disappointed that she would never be able to have biological children, but she wanted a dog, not kids! Doctors told Georgiann's mother the truth and not the fictitious lies about cancerous ovaries, but they simultaneously instructed her to go along with their lies and warned her that if Georgiann ever learned she had CAIS, the development of Georgiann's gender identity would forever be disrupted. These lies and this line of thinking are common throughout intersex medical practice (e.g., Karkazis), although perhaps to a lesser extent today (Davis). Years went by before Georgiann would uncover the medical lies and come to the realization that her mother was so upset at the time of diagnosis because doctors were forcing her to keep the intersex diagnosis from her daughter.

Doctors told Georgiann when she was diagnosed that she would have to have her cancerous ovaries, which were really healthy testes,[2] removed soon after she turned seventeen years old. Given what we know about the symbolic importance ovaries play in the construction of a women's gender identity (Elson), this news was traumatic on its own, aside from the cancer claims. When Georgiann looks back on this experience, she is surprised that she did not wonder why doctors would allow her to live with cancerous ovaries for years before removing them. But given she grew up in a working-class family, it makes sense that she did not think it was appropriate to question her doctors. Not long after Georgiann's seventeenth birthday, doctors rolled her into the operating room to surgically hide their lies by removing her healthy testes.

Georgiann remembers the open abdominal surgery as being incredibly physically painful. The pain still lives with her today, only now it surfaces as emotional pain and anger towards her doctors for subjecting her to genital mutilation. When Georgiann was in her early twenties, she had moved from her childhood healthcare providers. Under the assumption she had ovarian cancer as a teenager, she thought she would be proactive and request her medical records and bring them with her to her new doctor's office for a routine physical. As she walked to her car with the manila envelope filled with her medical records in her hands, she had no idea her life was about to forever change with the uncovering of medical lies.

As to be expected, Georgiann was curious about what doctors had written about her in her medical records. As she began to read through them, she was taken aback by the countless places where text was redacted with a black marker. But she did not let the redaction deter her. She held the medical records up to the bright sunny sky and read through the lies. She learned she was intersex, and although she immediately felt confused, followed by shock and even fear of her own body and medical history, she garnered the strength to read through every medical record—searching the internet for more explanation about what she was reading. Georgiann was initially scared to approach her parents with questions. She was concerned they would be hurt or angry that she found out the truth. Instead, she started her process of self-learning. She also did not feel she could trust her childhood doctors given they were never forthcoming with information about her intersex trait. At that time, she did not believe that any doctor was trustworthy, having been lied to by medical professionals for years. Many intersex people share similar narratives, and like Georgiann, they have had to learn about their intersex trait from sociocultural scholars and intersex activists and not the doctors who surgically mutilated their bodies (see Davis; Holmes; Karkazis; Kessler, "Medical Construction of Gender"; Preves).

Doctors got it wrong. When Georgiann learned about her intersex trait by uncovering the medical lies, her gender identity was not disrupted. Instead, like countless other intersex people (see Preves), she was angry with doctors for not leaving her body intact, for lying to her, and for encouraging her parents to go along with their lies. Although

Georgiann is an out intersex scholar activist today empowered by her intersex trait, she is left wondering how her life would have been different if doctors had not forced her to live in a body surgically shaped by medical lies. Would she be more trusting of medical professionals? Would her sexual desires be different?

Postsurgical (Pseudo) Menopause

It was during a fifth-grade English class that one of Georgiann's best friends got her period for the first time. Having not yet had any formal discussion of menstruation in school or at home, Georgiann had a lot of questions for her friend, such as "Is it painful?" and "How much are you bleeding?" Georgiann's friend answered the questions the best she could, but her answers left Georgiann hoping she would never get her period. Little did Georgiann know, her wish would be granted.

It's an unusual experience navigating the world as a young woman who never menstruated, especially given that for some girls and women menstruation is empowering (Fingerson; Lee). Georgiann did not want her period, per se, but she did mourn the inability to have biological children. As a young adult, Georgiann regularly felt uncomfortable when her friends talked about their menstrual cramps, their preference for pads or tampons, and their experiences concerning hormonal birth control (see Rodin for a discussion of the social construction of premenstrual syndrome). But she managed, and she did so by explaining to her friends what the doctors had told her—that she was in postsurgical menopause because of cancerous ovaries that needed to be removed. Her well-intended friends often downplayed Georgiann's experience saying things like, "Oh, you're sooooo lucky you don't get your period!" or, worse, "I will have a baby for you!" These words of support were harmful because they were not truthful. Later in life, when she learned it might have been possible for her to have biological children with in vitro fertilization if doctors had not removed her testes, she replaced the sadness due to her infertility with anger towards her medical professionals.

Although Georgiann was not initially bothered by never getting her period, she was still forced to experience pseudo-menopause under a medical lens—an experience shared by many intersex people (see Davis; Karkazis; Preves). After doctors removed Georgiann's testes, the primary producers of sex hormones in her body, they explained to her that she was, at seventeen years old, in postsurgical menopause. Given she never had a period, and menopause marks the permanent end of menstruation, doctors fabricated a faulty narrative by redefining menopause and, by default, menstruation. Yet because she did know the truth about her body, Georgiann believed she was in postsurgical menopause.

She was placed on a costly prescription estrogen patch—that never stayed on—to minimize the alleged effects that low levels of estrogen can have on the body, most notably issues pertaining to bone health (Mac Pherson; Gallagher) and sexual desire (Oudshoorn). Although there are differing opinions on the best course of action to address the bone health of intersex people who were subjected to the removal of their internal sex organs as children or teenagers ("Talk with Your Doctor"), we are compelled to ask the following: Would the issue of hormones and bone health be as big a concern for intersex people if their bodies were left intact? Although the relationship between sex hormonal levels and sexual desires is poorly understood, the correlation, for better or worse, is widely accepted by the general public as well as medical providers (Fausto-Sterling, *Myths of Gender*; Oudshoorn). Doctors explained to Georgiann that the hormone patch would provide her with the same amount of estrogen that other women of her age had in their bodies.

Medically described as being in postsurgical menopause, intersex people often feel the need to follow through with a doctor's recommendation for HRT. Doctors strongly recommend HRT for intersex people who were subjected to medically unnecessary and irreversible surgeries (e.g., Karkazis), despite a lack of evidence conclusively documenting its benefit in either intersex people or "normal" menopausal females (Lupton). HRT is costly, even for those with adequate health insurance, not to mention those who are uninsured or underinsured. While other girls and women are conveniently[3] purchasing pads and/or tampons, intersex people the same age have to buy expensive estrogen patches. Aside from the cost of HRT, doctors also do not know the right hormone regimen for intersex people. Do they even need HRT? How much estrogen should intersex people be on? Why estrogen and not testosterone or some combination of each? The answers to these questions are unclear, but what is clear is that we would not need to ask these questions if intersex people's bodily autonomy were respected and their bodies left intact. When doctors respond to intersex bodies by removing the primary producers of sex hormones as they do in most cases, they simultaneously establish the need for such questions about HRT and perpetuate assumptions about the relationship between sex hormones and normalcy.

As feminist scholar Nelly Oudshoorn documents, we often wrongly accept hormones as sex markers, where testosterone is associated with males and estrogen is associated with females. When doctors labeled Georgiann as experiencing postsurgical menopause, they were further perpetuating sex binary ideologies that maintain that people are biologically either neatly male or female (e.g., Fausto-Sterling, *Sexing the Body*; Fausto-Sterling, *Myths of Gender*; Kessler, "Medical Construction of Gender"). These are the same ideologies that prompted doctors to remove Georgiann's testes in the first place, and now doctors evoke these same ideologies in an attempt to script her gender hormonally with estrogen in order to maintain the arbitrary correlation between sex and gender. Because folks with CAIS, the intersex trait Georgiann has, appear externally female, doctors exclusively prescribe estrogen as HRT and ignore the fact that both estrogen and testosterone are found across all female bodies. In other words, in the minds of doctors, it is not appropriate to prescribe testosterone for those living with a female body (e.g., Fausto-Sterling, *Sexing the Body*).

Georgiann was never in postsurgical menopause. Rather, it is our assumption that doctors constructed her situation as synonymous with menopause to minimize the severity of their actions—the removal of her testes and the lies they told her about having ovarian cancer. In this way, we believe doctors drew on a biomedically defined status— postsurgical menopause—to create a narrative that made it seem as if they were helping, not harming, Georgiann. However, any hormonal deficiency that may exist in Georgiann's body, either today or in the future, is not a result of a natural hormonal problem; instead, it is due to doctors removing her internal testes because they refuse to recognize and acknowledge intersex people as human beings. This experience, which is all too common among intersex people (e.g., Preves), speaks to both the fluidity of social diagnoses (Jutel) and the power medical doctors have in the construction of medical diagnoses.

Conclusion: Patches Not Pads

This blended autoethnographic and life history account of Georgiann's intersex experience exemplifies how menopause is a socially constructed phenomenon. It also illustrates the power embedded with medicalization processes that leaves many individuals at the mercy of problematic doctors. After doctors removed Georgiann's testes, they labelled her as in postsurgical menopause to simultaneously minimize the human rights violation they enacted on her body and to reinforce sex and gender ideologies that maintain each as binary and correlated phenomenon (Kessler, "Medical Construction of Gender"). The fact that they apply the label without any reservation to an XY intersex female body that has never menstruated is remarkable, not only because of the person's anatomy but also because it highlights how the definition of menopause does not work in real life on real people. Such labelling also illustrates the power doctors have in controlling and perpetuating the definition of menopause (see also Bell, "Changing Ideas: The Medicalization of Menopause").

The example of trans women is different. Doctors do not label trans women, those who have transitioned from male to female, as being in menopause when they prescribe trans women exogenous estrogen. Instead, they describe trans women as being on medications to help them transition (see Davis, Dewey, and Murphy). Doctors have the power to "normalize" a trans woman's experience with hormones, and in life more generally, by using the medical language of menopause when referring to and treating trans women. For example, we can consider how menopause might be a gender-affirming label for trans women. Many doctors fail to offer gender-affirming healthcare (Gridley et al.), perhaps because they are more concerned with maintaining their medical authority, jurisdiction over bodies, and the perpetuation of sex and gender hegemonic ideologies than they are with affirming a trans woman's gender identity (Johnson; Sumerau and Mathers). Yet without hesitation, doctors often label intersex people who were subjected to medically unnecessary and irreversible interventions as being in postsurgical menopause (e.g., Preves). Perhaps doctors draw on menopause language after they perform medically unnecessary, irreversible, and nonconsensual surgical interventions on intersex people in order to justify their decision to label, and surgically shape, most intersex people as women. In the case of trans women, however, they do not need to justify any medical services they provide, for it is trans women who seek out their services. It would be interesting to explore whether or not doctors use menopause terminology in relation to the hormonal experiences of trans men. Given that most doctors hold strict ideologies about binary sex, it is likely they do use such language in exam rooms and in patients' charts when treating trans men, most likely to the disappointment of trans men who would likely prefer language that was more gender affirming (see Rydström). Although these assumptions are probable, they are best left to empirical analyses of the lived experiences of trans men.

We are not here to be the final arbiters of definitions of menopause, but we do feel compelled to hold doctors accountable for their attempt at being the constructors of both intersex and menopause status. Doctors should not surgically shape intersex people's bodies in order to force them into arbitrary sex and gender binaries. Nor should doctors feel empowered to impose a menopausal label on an intersex person in order to "normalize" the violation they enacted when they disrespected the person's bodily autonomy. Most intersex people will never menstruate, and, thus, they will never need pads. And they would not need hormonal patches either if doctors allowed intersex people to live in the bodies they were born in. We fear future generations of intersex people will continue to live their lives relying on patches and not pads, when they would be just fine without either.

Endnotes

1. Founded in 1993 by Cheryl Chase and other intersex activists, the Intersex Society of North America's purpose was two-fold: raise intersex visibility and encourage doctors to stop performing cosmetic surgeries on intersex people without their consent. In 2008, the Intersex Society of North America closed its doors. Its website remains active for historical record: www.isna.org/faq/conditions.

2. Georgiann's pathology results reveal that her testes were healthy and in no way cancerous. Medical research also overwhelmingly shows that those with CAIS have healthy testes (Nakhal et al.)

3. We feel it is important to note that pads and tampons can also be unduly expensive, which has has been recently demonstrated by activists around the globe protesting against the "tampon tax"—

the broad term that has been used to refer to sales taxes, value added taxes, and luxury taxes levied on menstrual hygiene products (Crawford and Spivack).

Works Cited

Bell, Susan E. "Sociological Perspectives on the Medicalization of Menopause." *Multidisciplinary Perspectives on Menopause. Annals of the New York Academy of Sciences.* Volume 592, edited by Marcha Flint, Fredi Kronenberg, and Wulf Utian, New York Academy of Sciences, 1990, pp. 173-78.

Bell, Susan E. "Changing Ideas: The Medicalization of Menopause." *Social Science & Medicine,* vol. 24, no. 6, 1987, pp. 535-42.

Blackless, Melanie, et al. "How Sexually Dimorphic Are We? Review and Synthesis." *American Journal of Human Biology,* vol. 12, no. 2, 2000, pp. 151-66.

Committee on Genetics: Section on Endocrinology and Section on Urology. "Evaluation of the Newborn with Developmental Anomalies of the External Genitalia." *Pediatrics,* vol. 106, no. 1, 2000, pp. 138-42.

Crawford, Bridget J. and Carla Spivack. "Tampon Taxes, Discrimination, and Human Rights." *Wisconsin Law Review,* vol. 3, 2017, pp. 491-549.

Crawley, Sara L. "Autoethnography as Feminist Self-Interview." *The Sage Handbook of Interview Research: The Complexity of Craft,* edited by Jaber F. Gubrium, et al., Sage, 2012, pp. 143-60.

Davis, Georgiann. *Contesting Intersex: The Dubious Diagnosis.* New York University Press, 2015.

Davis, Georgiann and Ellen Feder. "Normalizing Intersex." *Narrative Inquiry in Bioethics,* vol. 5, no. 2, 2015, pp. 87-89.

Davis, Georgiann, Jodie Dewey, and Erin L. Murphy. "Giving Sex: Deconstructing Intersex and Trans Medicalization Practices." *Gender & Society,* vol. 30, no. 3, 2016, pp. 490-514.

Dollard, John. *Criteria for the Life History, with Analysis of Six Notable Documents.* Yale University Press, 1935.

Dreger, Alice D., ed. *Intersex in the Age of Ethics.* University Publishing Group, 1999.

Elson, Jean. "Hormonal Hierarchy: Hysterectomy and Stratified Stigma. *Gender & Society*, vol. 17, no. 5, 2003, pp. 750-70.

Fausto-Sterling, Anne. *Sexing the Body: Gender Politics and the Construction of Sexuality.* New York: Basic Books, 2000.

Fausto-Sterling, Anne. *Myths of Gender: Biological Theories about Women and Men.* Basic Books, 1985.

Fingerson, Laura. *Girls in Power: Gender, Body, and Menstruation in Adolescence.* SUNY Press, 2006.

Gallagher, Christopher, J. "Effect of Early Menopause on Bone Mineral Density and Fractures." *Menopause*, vol. 14, no. 3, 2007, pp. 567-71.

Gridley, Samantha J., et al. "Youth and Caregiving Perspectives on Barriers to Gender-Affirming Health Care for Transgender Youth." *Journal of Adolescent Health*, vol. 59, 2016, pp. 254-61.

Hasson, Katie Ann. "Not a 'Real' Period? Social and Material Constructions of Menstruation." *Gender & Society*, vol. 30, no. 6, 2016, pp. 958-83.

Holmes, Morgan. *Intersex: A Perilous Difference.* Susquehanna University Press, 2008.

Johnson, Austin H. "Normative Accountability: How the Medical Model Influences Transgender Identities and Experiences." *Sociology Compass*, vol. 9, no. 9, 2015, pp. 803-13.

Jutel, Annemarie. *Putting a Name to It: Diagnosis in Contemporary Society.* Johns Hopkins University Press, 2014.

Karkazis, Katrina. *Fixing Sex: Intersex, Medical Authority, and Lived Experience.* Duke University Press, 2008.

Kessler, Suzanne J. *Lessons from the Intersexed.* Rutgers University Press, 1998.

Kessler, Suzanne J. "The Medical Construction of Gender: Case Management of Intersexed Infants." *Signs: Journal of Women in Culture and Society*, vol. 16, no. 1, 1990, pp. 3-26.

Lee, Janet. "Menarche and the (Hetero)Sexualization of the Female Body." *Gender & Society*, vol. 8, no. 3, 1994, pp. 343-62.

Lee, Peter A., et al. "Consensus Statement on Management of Intersex Disorders." *Pediatrics*, vol. 118, no. 2, 2006, pp. 488-500.

Leng, Kwok Wei. "On Menopause and Cyborgs: Or, rowards a Feminist Cyborg Politics of Menopause." *Body & Society*, vol. 2, no. 3, 1996, pp. 33-52.

Lupton, Deborah. "Constructing the Menopausal Body: The Discourses on Hormone Replacement Therapy." *Body & Society*, vol. 2, no. 1, 1996, pp. 91-97.

MacPherson, Kathleen I. "Osteoporosis and Menopause: A Feminist Analysis of the Social Construction of a Syndrome." *Advances in Nursing Science*, vol. 7, no. 4, 1985, pp. 11-22.

Morin, E. D. "Man with a Vagina." *Writing Menopause: An Anthology of Fiction, Poetry and Creative Nonfiction*, edited by Jane Cawthorne and E. D. Morin, Inanna Publications and Education, Inc., 2017, pp. 51-55.

Nakhal, Rola S., et al. "Evaluation of Retained Testes in Adolescent Girls and Women with Complete Androgen Insensitivity Syndrome." *Radiology*, vol. 268, no. 1, 2013, pp. 153-60.

Obermeyer, Carla Makhlouf. "Menopause Across Cultures: A Review of the Evidence." *Menopause*, vol. 7, no. 3, 2000, pp. 184-92.

Oudshoorn, Nelly. *Beyond the Natural Body: An Archeology of Sex Hormones.* Routledge, 1994.

Preves, Sharon. *Intersex and Identity: The Contested Self.* Rutgers University Press, 2003.

Rodin, Mari. "The Social Construction of Premenstrual Syndrome." *Social Science & Medicine*, vol. 35, no. 1, 1992, pp. 49-56.

Rydström Klara. "Degendering Menstruation: Making Trans Menstruators Matter." *The Palgrave Handbook of Critical Menstruation Studies*, edited by Chris Bobel, Inga T. Winkler, Breanne Fahs, Katie Ann Hasson, Elizabeth Arveda Kissling, and Tomi-Ann Roberts, Palgrave Macmillan, 2020, pp. 945-960.

Sumerau, J. E., and Lain A. B. Mathers. *America through Transgender Eyes.* Rowman & Littlefield, 2019.

"Talk with Your Doctor about HRT." *ISNA*, 2008, www.isna.org/faq/hrt_sousa. Accessed 5 Mar. 2021.

Warren, Carol A.B. "Gender Reassignment Surgery in the 18th Century: A Case Study." *Sexualities*, vol. 17, no. 7, 2014, pp. 872-84.

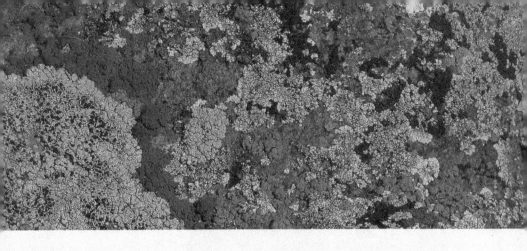

SECTION THREE
BLOOD RELATIONS

Wherein relationships of various kinds—mother and daughter,
woman and partner, women helping women—influence
perception, identity, decision making, and
sense of community throughout the transition to menopause.

Chapter 10

Waiting for
Seventeen Days

Heather Dillaway

S eventeen days late. My period hadn't been that late since I was training for cross-country in high school and, of course, when I was pregnant with my two children.

It was April 2018, and my daughter had just gotten her period for the first time. She wanted to download an app to start tracking her period, and she wanted me to download it, too. How fun, I thought! I had always just tracked and charted my period by placing an asterisk on a paper calendar because that's how my mom did it. The idea that my daughter and I would start tracking our periods together, simultaneously by app for the first time, was exciting in some strange way. I downloaded the app and was ready to use it. I knew my period would come in one week.

But it didn't come. Having studied menopause and reproductive aging for almost two decades, and having no other reason to miss a period that month, and having already experienced some early signs of peri-menopause, I knew the reason why my period was late. I have interviewed enough perimenopausal women to know exactly how periods start to shift and change and skip. But having a forty-seven-day cycle out of the blue was like being thrown off course, forced to miss the thirty-day mark my body and I were used to. And the most jarring part of the lateness was that I had been looking forward to using the period-tracking app with my daughter. I was almost ashamed to tell her I had nothing to track. Being seventeen days late that month meant being unlike her, when I thought we now were moving in parallel.

I have interviewed women who talked about comparing themselves to their teenaged daughters, but I did not know what that really felt like until that April. Somehow being late made me realize exactly how different my life stage is from my daughter's. What I thought was going to be an experience of sameness, of tracking together, was an experience of difference—her tracking and me *waiting*.

Waiting took me back to a blog post[1] I wrote in October 2010, in which I dug deeply into the idea of how waiting permeates much of women's reproductive experience:

> I have a friend who is "still waiting" for her menstrual cycle to be "normal" again after her second child and several other friends who are either "waiting" to figure out whether they will get pregnant, "waiting" to be done with their pregnancies, or "waiting" before they can have their last and final kid.... I started thinking more about how the menopausal women I interview always talk about "waiting" to figure out whether they are really "at menopause," or "waiting" to figure out if this is really their last menstrual period. Or how so many girls/young women who are sexually active are "waiting" to get their periods so that they can be relieved to know they are not pregnant. Or how women with painful periods, endometriosis, or migraines are waiting until those days are over each month. What does all of this reproductive waiting (waiting for menstruation, waiting for menstruation to be over, waiting for pregnancy, waiting for birth, waiting for menopause) mean?

> In all of these instances of reproductive waiting, waiting has a negative connotation and that seems to stem from the fact that we do not feel in control or in charge of our current reproductive time. When I think of the other situations in which I might use the word "waiting," the same holds true. I tell my kids to "wait their turn," and they don't like it. And none of us really like waiting in line. Fast food restaurants, frozen dinners, and ATM machines are all in existence because we don't have time or don't like to wait. Phrases that we use like "worth the wait" also connote negativity about waiting.

That April, when my period was seventeen days late, I was also *waiting*, and it felt negative. In writing that post in 2010, I explored several dictionary definitions of waiting, not all of which assumed negativity. But most defined "waiting" as a passive activity in which we remain, as one online source put it, "inactive in one place while expecting something." That was exactly what I felt like last spring. That was why those seventeen days felt so long to me. I felt forced to wait for something that I had expected would happen like clockwork.

Because my daughter was waiting for me to be able to use the app with her, we were both waiting. The waiting did lead to conversations about perimenopause. We had already talked a lot about menarche because it was important to me that she was not afraid and knew what to do when it happened. I also wanted her to be ready to think positively about her period. Before she was even able to understand what menstruation was, I called it the "good blood" so that she would come to understand her period as a sign of normality and good health.[2] But I had not told her much about perimenopause. I had not realized I would begin to have longer or irregular cycles so soon—at least it felt too soon. Then again, when I stopped to think about what I knew through my work and my research, I accepted that my perimenopause was right on time. So, I told her about it and about how natural and normal it was for me to start having strange and irregular cycles, even though I was not quite ready for this irregularity. We did not discuss my waiting every day, but I told her when I finally got my period.

My daughter has come to understand that both our menstrual lives are shifting, mine winding down while hers winds up. At least we have this shift in common. I reflect back on my own mother's perimenopause experiences, and I remember how frazzled and uncertain she seemed about her changes. Although we did not talk about it, I know now that waiting causes feelings of uncertainty. My mother had always been so sure of her reproductive trajectory until perimenopause, purposely having five kids, purposely birthing her kids at home, purposely teaching me to be in control of my own body. But the waiting at menopause startled her, too. Only now do I begin to understand how she must have felt about the uncertainty.

I thought a lot about the uncertainty of reproductive aging when I wrote the blog post about waiting. My late period added another layer to my own waiting experiences. All of this makes me think further about the uncertainty and impatience that women feel while waiting on menstruation or menopause or other reproductive events and whether it is actually the waiting (and not knowing) that makes women feel negative about their experiences.

I think again about the word—"waiting"—and I wonder about the heaviness and negativity of this word. Maybe the word itself is the problem. I saw myself as passively waiting for my period, just like many women do. As commenters on my blog post suggested, the word itself connotes a sense of powerlessness. I also described waiting in my blog post as akin to feeling out of control. Other words, like "tracking," feel more empowering as they allow women the chance to involve themselves in their own reproductive life courses—to record, observe, chart, follow, and participate in their reproductive events and experiences.[3] Perhaps I need to adjust the way I'm thinking about the ongoing irregularity of my periods and be more mindful of the observing and tracking that I can do instead of just waiting and remaining uncertain as I navigate perimenopause. I can remain an active participant in this life stage and show my daughter that we can live in our moments, however confusing they sometimes can be.

I was waiting that April. I was impatient. I wanted to be able to track my period like I had in previous months and do it alongside my daughter. When I was seventeen days late, it felt as if something had been stolen from me. I have thought a lot about why I was so bothered by my lateness that month and decided it was about my desire to connect and share experiences with my daughter. We anticipated her menarche but neither of us completely minded this wait—it did not feel that negative, and we knew her period would come when her body was ready. I could have applied the same outlook when looking ahead to irregular cycles, something I was not actively anticipating that year but could have been. I could have engaged my daughter in active tracking and charting of my upcoming late period so that she would learn from me that attention, observation, and tracking are positive at every juncture. Passive waiting was not the only option. It is interesting what you learn in retrospect.

I have been able to connect with my daughter in many ways in the months since, but the co-incidence of her menarche and my peri-menopausal event was clarifying. The experience of my own waiting, not tracking or charting, awoke me to the differences in our reproductive events and made me more mindful of my personal reproductive path. Acknowledging that my perimenopause has begun means learning to adapt to a different kind of tracking and charting experience. This new stage of waiting and tracking will not look like my daughter's or my previous waiting or tracking, even though there will be similarities at times. She is adjusting to unexpected heavy bleeding and so am I, so we can compare notes about this and other bodily signs and changes, maybe just not by calendar day. Actively monitoring and knowing when the heavy bleeding might come, for instance, is useful for both us so that we are prepared to alleviate or manage it with extra supplies at hand.

As we approach the third anniversary of tracking our cycles together, my daughter and I have fallen into a regular pattern of casual conversation about the use of the app, reports on her friends' menarches, the signs of our own upcoming periods, and how to deal with uncomfortable or inconvenient bodily moments. Even though my daughter's early periods have been somewhat irregular, as expected, she is now adjusting to cyclicity and regularity as I am adjusting to irregularity. We are now aware of the different courses we are tracking and charting in the app we downloaded, but there is comfort and unity in adjusting to our new life stages together.

Endnotes

1. My post "Waiting" appeared on *Menstruation Matters*, the blog of the Society for Menstrual Cycle Research, on Oct. 28, 2010: www. menstruationresearch.org/2010/10/28/waiting/.

2. I told both my daughter and my son about the "good blood" early on and wrote about this topic for *Menstruation Matters*.

3. I thank the commenters on my blog post who encouraged me to think less passively about this topic.

Works Cited

"Waiting." *Collins English Dictionary—Complete and Unabridged*, 2014, www.thefreedictionary.com/waiting. Accessed 5 Mar. 2021.

Dillaway, Heather. "Sorry, You'll Never Get the Good Blood..." *Menstruation Research*, 6 June 2012, www.menstruationresearch.org/2012/06/21/sorry-you'll-never-get-the-good-blood.../. Accessed 5 Mar. 2021.

Dillaway, Heather. "Waiting." *Menstruation Research*, 28 Oct. 2010, www.menstruationresearch.org/2010/10/28/waiting/. Accessed 5 Mar. 2021.

Chapter 11

"Dear Magnolia... Nobody Really Understands... What Can I Do?" Reflections on a Perimenopausal Blog as Social Support

Gillian Anderson

Sleepless nights, exhaustion, irritability, night sweats, acne, bra rage, hot flashes, forgetfulness. What is a perimenopausal woman to do? Conventional wisdom suggests women experiencing perimenopause often confide in and rely on their relations with other women, friends, families, social support networks, and/or chosen healthcare providers to make their way through this so-called change of life (Duffy, Iversen, and Hannaford 561). Ethnographic data reveal perimenopausal women may seek out both lay persons and experts, favouring "personal experts" or those "deemed professionally sound and personally relevant" (Thompson) to assist them through the transition. However, in the age of social media, individuals are also increasingly and regularly seeking out health-related information from a range of online sources (Tonsaker, Bartlett and Trpkov 407).[1] A growing number of studies on online support groups dedicated to women's health issues—most notably breast cancer (Elder and Burke; Orgad; Seale; Seale, Ziebland and Charteris-Black; Vilhauer), depression (Kotliar), multiple sclerosis (Sosnowy), eating disorders (Eichorn), and body image (Turner)—attest to this trend. Studies focused on women's reproductive health also include research on pregnancy (Fredricksen, Harris, and Moland; Johnson; Ley; Nolan et al.), pregnancy loss (Gold, Normandin, and Boggs), breastfeeding (Brown, Raynor, and Lee; Cowie, Hill and Robinson), postpartum depression (Teaford, Goyal, and McNiesh), and aging (Im et al.; Trudeau et al.).

The menopausal transition represents a natural stage of women's reproductive aging (Soules et al.). Interestingly as of March 2016, a search of "online support groups" in sociological abstracts returns some 541 results, yet "online support groups and menopause" only returns two. Of these, one considers how numerous changes over women's life course, including but not limited to menopause, are "negotiate[d]" by the giving and receiving of support through "mediated communication channels" (Dare and Green 270), whereas the other focuses on women's decision making surrounding hormone therapy (Sillence et al.). A search for "online support groups and perimenopause" returns zero results. To date, it appears sociologists have not empirically examined online menopause support groups, not to mention perimenopausal blogs, which is surprising in light of the aforementioned findings and the prevalence of social media.

In this chapter, I present an exploratory, qualitative content analysis of a North American perimenopause blog. My narrative analysis of select blog entries (n=86), archived between June 2014 and March 2016, contributes to the "talk among women" embraced by this edited collection. I suggest blog entries embody a metanarrative that centres women's desire for a supportive community during perimenopause. Embedded in this overarching narrative are three "carrying themes" (Hall and Powell) or types of perimenopausal talk, the first of which I refer to as "transitional talk." By "transitional talk," I mean talk that characterizes perimenopause as a tumultuous but temporary and transitional time in women's lives. The women's narratives also voice what I term "symptom speak"—narratives that talk about the experience and management of perimenopausal symptoms. And, lastly, the women's narratives articulate what I call "support speak," which entails the solicitation and provision of social support that is narratively "co-constructed" (Hall and Powell) by both blogger and readers alike. Informational and emotional supports

(Koch and Mansfield) figure prominently in women's support speak. My thematic analysis illustrates how the sharing of personal narratives enhances our understanding of the menopausal transition and the significance of blogs as an underresearched yet potentially important social support mechanism for perimenopausal women's socio-emotional wellbeing.

Social Support and Perimenopausal Women

The concept of social support refers to "any process through which social relationships may promote health and well-being" (Cohen, Underwood, and Gottlieb 4). Supports may be emotional, informational, and/or instrumental (Koch and Mansfield 179). Communicative (Mattson and Gibb Hall) and interactive (Dare and Green; Gottlieb; Rains and Keating) processes are also noted in the literature. Marifran Mattson and Jennifer Gibb Hall conceptualize social support "as a transactional communicative process, including verbal and/or nonverbal communication that aims to improve an individual's feelings of coping, competence, belonging, and/or esteem" (184). Benjamin Gottlieb, meanwhile, defines social support largely as "the process of interaction in relationships which improves coping, esteem, belonging and competence through actual or perceived exchanges of physical or psychosocial resources" (qtd. in Mattson and Gibb Hall 183).

Social support is an important part of women's day-to-day lives (Dare and Green 486), which may be especially true for middle-aged women whose lives are characterized by transition and change (Bresnahan and Murray Johnson qtd. in Dare and Green 475). Empirically, the support of family, friends, and medical professionals has been found to be key in helping women navigate perimenopause (Duffy, Iversen, and Hannaford). Women's relations with friends (Duffy, Iverson, and Hannaford), family (Dillaway, "Menopause"; Duffy, Iverson, and Hannaford), husbands (Mansfield, Koch, and Gierach), and intimate partners (Dillaway "Why Can't You Control This?") have been investigated, as have relations with healthcare providers (Baird), including the role of healthcare providers in normalizing the management of menopause (Thompson). For instance, more than 60 per cent of Scottish women aged forty-five to fifty-four in a community-based study reported talking to family and friends as a major form of social support accessed in their attempts to deal with menopausal symptoms, with friends being perceived as "the most supportive" (Duffy, Iverson, and Hannaford 560). The study found approximately 20 per cent of women wished their spouse or partners were more supportive, whereas almost 40 per cent expressed wanting more support from their family doctor or practice nurse (554, 560). Relatedly, research has revealed that some husbands socially support their wives, but others feel ill-equipped, citing a lack of information or assuredness and/or having to deal with middle-age stressors themselves (Mansfield, Koch, and Gierach 109).

Some research suggests women not only need to be able to access various types of support from their existing social networks, but may also have to cultivate new networks and engage professional help to aid in the process of finding effective menopausal management strategies (Koch and Mansfield 179). However, women's ability to access information and supportive decision-making options may be marked by stratification and inequality (Thompson). Studies show racial and ethnic differences in how women experience and make sense of menopause (Dillaway, "Menopause"; Im et al.) and perimenopause (Reece and Harkless). Differential access to treatment along the lines of race and social class have also been found to exist (Dillaway, "Menopause").

In short, women are apt to pursue a variety of lay and expert resources in their attempts to manage menopause (Thompson). Increasingly, social media may be a resource; thus, scholars have begun to investigate the giving and receiving of social support online (Coulson and Knibb; Coulson; Coulson, Buchanan, and Aubeeluck; Hong et al.; Letourneau et al.; Weinert, Cudney, and Winters; Weinert; White and Dorman). Studies of menopause and online social support are rare. Mary Jiang Bresnahan and Lisa Murray-Johnson's (2002) analyses of an internet-based health discussion group found that women came to rely on what they termed "a community of support" in order to help them deal with the changes associated with and to "make sense" of menopause (398). Julie Dare and Lelia Green have noted how women exchange social support in relation to changes experienced across the life course, including menopause, vis-a-vis email and online chat rooms. Social support via blogging has been less studied, and research on perimenopausal blogs at present seems nonexistent. My analysis of these personal yet public narratives reveals perimenopausal women's desire for connection and community and their pursuit and provision of social support online.

I centre their voices to understand the meanings women attach to their lived experiences and to illustrate how we might view blogging as "empowering" (Sosnowy) and/or online storytelling as a "socially meaningful activity" (Orgad 1), which affirms women's agency during this transitional time.

Online Social Support and Perimenopausal Blogs

Given the popularity of social media, it seems reasonable some perimenopausal women might turn to online sources of social support, including blogs. Blogs are a site of social interaction. They are characterized as "an online journal or informational website displaying information in the reverse chronological order, with latest posts appearing first ... where a writer or even a group of writers share their views on an individual subject" (Djuraskovic). This means a "blog author" posts a message, article, picture, or link to another website and leaves space below for readers to respond, comment, and ask questions (Hookway; Poore). Posts may be "archived allowing researchers to map the development of a theme through the conversations surrounding it" (Wilson, Kenny, and Dickson-Swift 2015).

Recent studies consider the possibilities and challenges blogs present for social and health researchers (Hookway; Wilson, Kenny, and Dickson). Prior research finds women tend to "personal" blog more than men in terms of the creation of "intimate and emotional" content (Pedersen and Macaffee qtd. in Kotliar 1205), emphasize disease and disability (Miller, Pole, and Bateman qtd. in Kotliar 1205), and value the "social interaction" or "social aspects of blogging" (Pedersen and Macaffee 1482). Some research suggests health blogging may "benefit those most in need of support" (Rains and Keating 529). According to Hsiu-Chia Ko, Li-Ling Wang, and Yi-Ting Xu, "The interactive or communicative process through which bloggers reveal their moods, everyday lives, experiences, or other information, as well as the audience responses posted in the comment box, can be considered an act of social support" (194). My analysis of a perimenopausal blog reflects what Sophia Alice Johnson refers to as the "changing nature of social support and information-seeking practices" (237), where blogs may be understood as "informal support resources" (Hunting 3).

Data and Method

The Perimenopause Blog: Yes, it's Real & No, You Aren't Going Crazy was founded in 2009 by Magnolia Miller, owner of Pink Zinnia Publishing & Health Communications. With a professional certification in healthcare consumer advocacy and a master's degree specializing in health communication and narrative medicine, this self-described freelance health and medical writer "is a passionate and loyal advocate for women who are struggling with hormone imbalance during perimenopause, but can't seem to get the help they need and want from the medical community"[2] ("About The Perimenopausal Blog"). In the menopause blogosphere, her blog is distinct in its focus on perimenopause. *Healthline*, a website that reportedly attracts 125 million visitors monthly, named *The Perimenopause Blog* the top menopause blog for three consecutive years (2016, 2017, and 2018). Magnolia's own website invites readers to join her "over 5000 monthly subscribers." In February 2019, *The Perimenopause Blog*'s Facebook page had over 5,700 likes and 5,564 followers.

The Perimenopause Blog is best described as a personal blog (Kotliar), as it "concern[s] personal, day-to-day, and even intimate issues that have to do with bloggers' private lives" (Hollenbaugh qtd. in Kotliar 1205). Magnolia openly shares her own personal narrative in the blog, including her struggles, frustrations, and desire to find a sympathetic ear so that she might better understand but also navigate what she characterizes as her "hormone-filled and bumpy ride through perimenopause" (Miller, "My [Hormone-Filled and Bumpy] Ride"). Magnolia notes that at her blog, readers "will find plenty of up-to-date articles, books, products, and a community of other women just like you who are sharing their stories" ("About the Perimenopause Blog"). When Magnolia started her blog, she intended to answer "any and all comments." Over time, the volume of reader "traffic and comments" made responding to everyone unwieldy. She remedied this by creating "Dear Magnolia," where she regularly features a reader comment or question (often crafted in the form of a letter) and then posts her reply and answers. She hopes readers with "similar complaints and questions" will collectively benefit from her "new venture" ("Archives," 5 June 2014). In this way, Magnolia initiates or structures the conversation around a particular topic or issue that she feels is "representative of what a lot of other women go through too" (9 Aug. 2014). Readers, in turn, join the dialogue to respond and comment, but they are also able to talk among themselves.

The "Dear Magnolia" archive is a rich source of data and of empirical interest. As of March 2016, it contained eighty-six entries, including Magnolia's featured posts, her and other readers' replies and comments. All entries (n=86) posted between June 2014 and March 2016 were retrieved, openly coded, and analyzed for this chapter.[3] Here, I share exemplary entries to anchor my analysis. Posts such as "Dear Magnolia... Nobody Really Understands... What Can I Do?," "Dear Magnolia... Not Every Woman Hates Their Husband in Perimenopause," and "Dear Magnolia... Does Anybody Really Give a Crap?" have elicited supportive responses from Magnolia and readers. The number of comments posted to each entry vary from a minimum of zero to a maximum of twenty-four. The average is eleven. The "Dear Magnolia... About that Vertigo and Dizziness in Perimenopause" post (August 2014) has elicited the most responses to date. Taken together, not only do these entries offer insight into how some women mediate this period of transition, but the sharing of these personal narratives also begs the question as to whether the blog itself may also be characterized as a meaningful social support network for both the blogger and readers alike, and its importance as a support strategy is worthy of consideration.

The Metanarrative of "Supportive Community"

A central and organizing narrative evident in "Dear Magnolia" is perimenopausal women's desire to connect with other women at this stage in their lives. They want someone to talk to, to listen, to relate to, and confide in. Someone they can share their feelings and experiences with. Women want support and are online actively creating or searching for a sense of community. One of the main "functions" (Coulson, Buchanan, and Aubeeluck 173) of *The Perimenopause Blog*, then, is its ability to act as a "supportive community." The blog brings women together in a shared space. It fosters connections, reduces feelings of social isolation, and provides opportunities for women to seek and offer support to one another. The importance of being a part of a supportive community during perimenopause is perhaps best voiced by a commenter named Found the Solution who comments:

> We all need a female friend (or two or three, like on this blog) to talk with. It's fine to pay a shrink, but there's no shrink like a

best buddy. Mountain climbers don't climb alone, divers, don't dive alone, and we shouldn't go through menopause alone…I recommend getting online and joining a 'meetup' group, if you need to make some friends. I hope sharing my own journey here gives others hope and encourages them in their quest to find a solution that works for them. (15 Oct. 2014)

Magnolia was so impressed with Found the Solution that she not only featured her story but sent her a personal thank you via email, saying she "encapsulates everything I have blogged about here at the Perimenopause Blog over the years" (15 Oct. 2014).

Women are relieved and overjoyed to have found this community. They repeatedly note how "helpful," "informative," "inspirational," "calming," and "comforting" it is. They express gratitude. Sarah, for example, posts: "Please help. Any advice is greatly appreciated as I have no one else to talk to about these issues. Everyone else just thinks they are in my head. Thanks Sarah" (4 Aug. 2014). Tammy says, "I am so relieved I found this site and this article … so I just keep reaching out and reading these articles and getting much relief knowing there are others like me" (24 June 2015). And Jennie comments: "I'm so happy to have found this post and comments by other women. I felt like I have been losing my mind for months! Someone tell me there is a light at the end of this tunnel. I've cancelled family vacations, I have found drivers for my kids soccer, and basically don't want to leave the house. I never thought I'd feel this way" (10 Oct. 2014).

Women are assured their feelings and experiences are "normal" or "real." "I am so happy to have found your blog. I feel like I am going crazy, but I know I am in perimenopause," says Angie (11 Dec. 2015). In response to Angie, Magnolia shares her rationale for starting the blog. She meant it to be a supportive space. Her post reassures Angie, among others, that women want and need an aforementioned "community of support":

One of the reasons I began this blog was to offer women like yourself a place of support, information, and reassurance that you're going to be okay. For me, and for most women I've found, just the simple assurance that what you're experiencing is "normal" as it were, does so much to ease the stress. You're going to be fine…. That's a promise … get thee over the Perimenopause Blog Facebook page where you will find lots of women just like you who can provide emotional support as well! And let me leave you with one final assurance that you're going to be fine! You're already taking the necessary steps to get this under control. That is the best, and frankly, all you can do at this point. And remember... this too shall pass! (1 Jan. 2016)

Moreover, perimenopausal women are seen to be agentic actors. Michelle's post explicitly locates women's agency in supportive conversations like these:

Hi Magnolia, Thanks for your quick response and validation. I am so happy that I found your blog and have found comfort and support in your story, as well as those of the many women who have and are experiencing symptoms of perimenopause and menopause. I hope to soon be able to report back with a positive outcome. There is power in women having open, honest and supportive conversations about their health and well-being. (3 Nov. 2015)

Women desire support and a supportive community in mediating the perimenopausal transition. "Dear Magnolia" affords women an online space for actively engaging in this social interaction. Online exchanges are crucial. They help combat feelings of isolation. That "Dear Magnolia" is a sought after and welcome space is evident in women's collective sense of relief having found the blog. *The Perimenopause Blog* acts as a social support network; it affirms, validates, and normalizes (Mattson and Gibb Hall) women's subjective experiences and narrative claims. Both Magnolia and her readers "seek and find mutual understanding, form social networks [and] share experience" (Sosnowy vi). Although the blog was started by Magnolia to support women like herself going through perimenopause, it may also be the case that readers' comments and posts enhance the health and wellbeing of her as the blogger, too. These may be interpreted as "intertwined activities," as a means of "self-therapy and helping others" (Huh et al. 8). This "interactive" (Dare and Green; Gottlieb; Rains and Keating) process may be interpreted not only as a meaningful, supportive activity but also as a way meaning and solidarity are co-constructed through shared and/or collective conversations. It is these "moving," "thoughtful," "intelligent," "enlightening," and "inspirational" conversations that are, according to Magnolia, "good for all of us."

Transitional Talk

Within this supportive community, posts reinforce the idea that perimenopause is a period of transition. This "transitional talk" is voiced by Magnolia and her readers. It is expressed explicitly and indirectly. Magnolia says, "Perimenopause is a transition period, not a life sen-tence" (5 June 2014). This theme is implied in her repetitive use of phrases, such as "Repeat as often as you need to: this too shall pass" (22 Aug. 2014) and "Let me assure you that all of the hormonal imbalance will pass" (5 June 2014). Magnolia tells Mandy: "Peri-menopause is a raucous ride and you just have to hang on with your might. What you are doing is helping, though it may not seem like it at times. Hang in there!" (3 Jan. 2016). Crazy Auntie describes peri-menopause as a "physiological transition ... if perimenopause is playing a part in your lives right now, please don't take it personally" (25 Nov. 2015). She says, "I have learned so much from your resources here and being able to refer back to them when times are tough is a big part of what keeps me assured that this transition will someday stabilize" (27 Nov. 2015). Angie echoes Magnolia's refrain, "This blog has helped to reassure me that this too shall pass" (1 Jan. 2016), to which Magnolia replies: "You're going to be fine. You will get through this, all of this 'crazy' eventually, and you will feel 'normal' again. That's a promise.... And remember this too shall pass."

Transitional talk may be interpreted in a number of ways. Perimenopause may be read as an in-between or liminal space. Whereas Lisa and Ann talk about themselves as being on the threshold of perimenopause—"I'm forty-three and perimenopausal, at least, I think I am" (Lisa) and "I am only thirty-nine! I know that's young to start perimenopause, or at the very young end" (Ann) (16 Oct. 2014)—Pam, age fifty-one, who has been in perimenopause for four years, thinks she has "hit bigtime perimenopause now" (25 Sept. 2015). Bobbi, age forty-three, who had a hysterectomy at twenty-eight, did not think she would have to "go through this lovely change" (24 June 2014). Crazy Auntie compares perimenopause to puberty. She notes the same awkwardness, but how adult responsibilities make keeping "it together" during "late stage perimenopause ... pure hell sometimes" (25 Nov. 2015).

Perimenopause is understood as a "journey" or "quest" that women "navigate." It signifies a passage of time but of varied or unknown duration. This is evident in the stories of women who have "survived" or made it "through." Lisa says, "even though I'm not convinced this will ever end, it helps to hear from women who've survived and are enjoying life on the other side." Responding to Lisa, Magnolia says: "Perimenopause means you are saying goodbye to the 'young you' and getting acquainted with a 'new you.' But it's not an easy introduction. You have to go through all of those other symptoms too—and it's not easy.... I've come to terms with moving past the years of reproduction. I have accepted that I am no longer the hot thirty-year-old I once was, and it's ok" (22 Aug. 2014).

These narratives reflect change, including changing bodies, social statuses, selves, or identities. Change may be tied to the loss of one's fertility and a reproductive self or to the emergence of a new sense of self, accompanied by greater self-awareness and acceptance. Michelle posts that "On September 15 [2015], I lost the old me" (5 Nov. 2015). In her reply, Magnolia reminds her of the following:

> Remember, also, that you will not be the "old me" anymore. You are changing. Your body is changing, and, therefore, you must allow these changes to occur. On the other side of perimenopause is menopause and a "new normal" and a "new me." Let that happen. Grieve the loss of what was if you need to, but embrace your life now, as it is. We can't go back. So, have to adapt, adjust and accept. (3 Nov. 2015)

Becky's post reiterates this idea:

> When I was perimenopausal, I truly didn't like who I had become. I was depressed, angry, tired, moody etc. I was doing and saying things that just weren't me. I was actually grieving the loss of my sensual sexual me, and I wasn't very happy about it.... But as Magnolia says, we have to go through it to get to the other side. We grow through the pain. It does not last forever and there is a light at the end of the tunnel. (24 Sept. 2014)

Transitional talk suggests perimenopause is a normal stage of life most women endure. Perimenopause is talked about as a tumultuous but temporary process. It reflects a passage of time, the length of which, though uncertain, is finite. Transitional talk articulates changes associated with women's reproductive aging, including physical changes and perceived changes in social status and identity. It highlights women's struggles to negotiate or navigate this in-between space and make sense of who they are, who they are no longer, and who they eventually become. Such talk eases women in the midst of perimenopause, enabling a self-described "wise sage" to conclude: "Menopause is actually quite liberating" (24 Sept. 2014).

Symptom Speak

Frequently, posts coalesce around a variety of perimenopausal symptoms, whether they are physical, socioemotional, or psychological. I refer to women's talk of symptoms and related difficulties as "symptom speak." The following exchange illustrates this theme. Mindy, struggling to deal with a range of symptoms, notes the following:

> First of all, I have to say I love this site! My question is as I find all the symptoms, confusing and a bit scary. I am forty-eight years old and have been having many of the symptoms ... it seems every night I go to bed, and I wake up drenched in sweat. I am not on fire like a furnace but slightly warm and sometimes cold and clammy. My forehead, neck, chest, stomach, arms, and armpits, and even sometimes part of my legs are wet. My pillow and sheets are also wet. I am wondering if there is something seriously wrong or could this be perimenopause? Is this hot flashes or night sweats? I never seem to have a good night sleep, as I am always waking up. I try to mention this to my [doctor], but he said he didn't think it's a hormonal thing. My sister told me it's all perimenopause. What do you think? And could you please tell me more about hot flashes and night sweats and such? I know this is all not in my head. I also get prickly skin or burning skin feeling all over. Thank you so much. (5 June 2014)

To which Magnolia replies:

Dear Mindy,

At the age of forty-eight you are not too young to be in perimenopause. So, as usual, I'm baffled as to why your doctor would tell you something as absurd as your night sweats and hot flashes are not hormonal. The first thing I would suggest is that you find a physician who has more knowledge of hormone imbalance in women. Hot flashes and night sweats during perimenopause are caused by the fluctuating estrogen levels….Your sister is correct to tell you what you are experiencing is perimenopause related—because it is…. And finally, please let me assure you that all of the hormonal imbalance will pass. Perimenopause is a transition period, not a life sentence. Once your hormones stabilize you will begin to feel better. Not all women choose to use hormone therapy to help with their symptoms. However, if you do, I would strongly recommend that you educate yourself and consider bioidentical hormone therapy over synthetic hormones. They are safer and have not been shown to pose any increased risk of breast cancer, stroke, or heart disease. (5 June 2014)

Symptom speak reveals perimenopausal women's expression of a range of emotions, including anger, rage, sadness, and despair. Grief and dealing with loss emerge in these emotion-laden narratives. Voicing the trouble she has articulating her grief, Lisa writes:

Hi Magnolia,

I just want to add my voice to the many women who've thanked you for sharing your experience and wisdom on this blog…. The hardest part is, I think, the grief. I go through bouts of anxiety and depression, but the grief is just constant. It's this sadness that just follows me everywhere. It's in every thought and everything I do. I have such a hard time explaining how I feel to people who have never been there…. Anyway, I just had to thank you. You've helped me keep what's left of my sanity. (22 Aug. 2016)

To which Magnolia reassuringly replies the following:

Dear Lisa,

Your comment touched me. I was in my early forties when I began to go through perimenopause too…. I remember feeling exactly the way you feel…. I've been in menopause for well over three years now…. I can assure you [that] you will feel less sad as you inch closer to menopause and [accept the] change. (22 Aug. 2014)

Conversations centred on symptoms are ones most women can readily relate to. At times, readers tend to appear to be more focused on their own subjective experiences (their symptoms and lives), yet they simultaneously relate and acknowledge a shared set of symptoms and collective experiences. Beyond allowing women to question or complain about their symptoms, "Dear Magnolia" acknowledges that these symptoms, though normal, can still be challenging and difficult. In "Dear Magnolia.... Nobody Really Understands... What Can I Do?" Magnolia describes a woman's symptoms as "typical" but also makes it clear "that in no ways diminishes how she is feeling." She suggests her symptoms are "'normal' even if they are making her feel as if she is going crazy" (1 Jan. 2016).

Magnolia and her readers speak of treatment options to help alleviate perimenopausal symptoms. Discussions of symptom management may be indicative of a more "informational" or "instrumental" (Koch and Mansfield) type of support as identified in the existing literature. Conversations about the pros and cons of bioidentical hormone therapy, including the relative success or failure of such therapy, are common. Whereas some women seem to seek a "quick fix," Magnolia herself notes: "Hormone therapy takes time. You can't pop a pill and magically fix everything" (1 Jan. 2016). The following exchange captures these ideas. In "Dear Magnolia... Bioidentical Hormones Have Worked for Me!" (15 Oct. 2014), Found the Solution notes the challenges in finding a knowledgeable healthcare provider, one who is responsive to women's individual needs and well versed on the subject of bioidentical hormone replacement therapy (BHRT). She encourages women to be persistent and proactive in searching out potential management options and stresses the importance of making informed decisions regarding their care and body. She advises women to educate and empower themselves. Women are afforded agency in this process:

> My feeling is that a woman needs to be proactive about her own health and well-being. My advice to women going through this process: empower and educate yourself; read books on BHRT and decide if it's a good option for you; If so, do some research and find out if various doctors prescribe BHRT—eventually you'll find one who will listen to you and respect your decisions regarding the care of your own body!! Since we are all individuals, adjusting and re-balancing hormones can take time, but most

women begin to feel 'more like themselves' pretty quickly.... I hope sharing my own journey gives others hope and encourages them in their quest to find a solution that works for them! (15 Oct. 2014)

In her reply, Magnolia praises taking on a proactive role to manage her experience:

Dear Found the Solution,

I can't thank you enough for your wonderful comment. I was delighted to read of your success and how much bioidentical hormones, exercise, diet, and a network of friends for emotional support has [sic] helped you navigate the crazy world of perimenopause.... I applaud your efforts to take personal responsibility for your health and wellbeing. It clearly paid off for you. And thank you again for sharing your wonderful story with the readers of the *Perimenopause Blog*.

Magnolia applauds readers' attempts to manage their perimenopausal symptoms in ways that work best for them as well as their willingness to share their experiences. Although these personal stories add value to the blog's community, they also hold the potential for personal bias. A critical reader must be mindful to differentiate between symptom speak centred on the provision of informational support and the promotion of certain treatments that may or may not be data based.

My analysis of symptom speak offers insight into how women talk about perimenopausal symptoms on the blog. "Dear Magnolia" is a supportive community for women to engage in open and frank discussions about symptoms and treatment options. Women voice their concerns and complaints, ask questions, and offer feedback to each other. While acknowledging their symptoms are real and normal, dealing or coping with these symptoms can also be hard. Symptom speak does not downplay, nor does it alleviate these problems; rather, it appears to reassure women they need not suffer alone or in silence. Engaging in symptom speak may make dealing with perimenopause more bearable.

Support Speak

Women pursue and provide social support via "Dear Magnolia." Informational and emotional support figure prominently in women's "support speak." The provision of informational social support is shown more often in Magnolia's posts, although readers occasionally offer their own helpful hints and advice as well. This support is demonstrated by Magnolia referring readers to an array of resources, including books, videos, products, or treatment possibilities. She cites articles on topics, such as hot flashes and night sweats, bioidentical estrogen, and hormone therapy. She shares links to diet and exercise regimes, including yoga and Pilates. Replying to Michelle's queries on vertigo and perimenopause, Magnolia includes links to articles on vertigo, dizziness, foggy thinking, and adrenal fatigue. She suggests an exercise video, embeds a hyperlink to an antihistamine, and recommends Dr. Christiane Northrup's book, *The Wisdom of Menopause.* She closes by saying she "hope[s] this helps Michelle, and answers [her] questions" (2 Aug. 2014). However, before Michelle responds, Cassie comments, "I hope you feel better soon, Michelle... Take care and best wishes!" (3 Aug. 2014). Valerie says: "Your story is my story Michelle. I'm in the perimenopause stage. I've had [v]ertigo for over a year now...I found a product at Walgreens called 'Vertigo.' It is a natural remedy you roll on the back of your neck during a [v]ertigo moment and it's helped me by relieving the symptoms quickly. Take care!" (3 Aug. 2014). Michelle then replies with thanks and says she plans to get the recommended book (8 Aug. 2014).

Relationships and emotional support are recurring themes in women's support speak. Women talk about these ideas in two ways. First, they talk about the perceived impact perimenopause has on their relationships, particularly their marriages. Strained relations, a lack of empathy, and communication difficulties are mentioned. They often lament their husband's inability to provide the type of support they need. K who describes herself as "in a hormonal shit storm with no avenue to open up dialogue" with her husband asks:

How do I talk to my husband about perimenopause? He seems to think I am exaggerating ailments and generally blames me for not being able to pull myself out of it.... I'm just tired physically, mentally, and emotionally. I'm starting to take care of me, but I've been met with resistance. How do I begin a dialogue about perimenopause without opening the door for blaming and resentment? (1 Dec. 2015)

Magnolia responds by suggesting that until K's husband is willing to realize that he is able to exert as much control over his hormones as K is of hers, such problems will likely persist. She apologizes for saying as much but says, "It is the truth. I hope, however, you can find some comfort and support here. And do join us on Facebook" (9 Dec. 2015). When talking about marriage, Magnolia speaks of her own as well as about her divorce. Her common refrain is that perimenopause is not the cause of marital conflict and or problems in a relationship per se. Perimenopause may, however, draw out or exacerbate preexisting or underlying marital issues. Magnolia's response to Julia, who shares her struggle to deal with a number of perimenopausal symptoms while contemplating a divorce, conveys this. In her post titled, "Dear Magnolia... Not Every Woman Hates Their Husband in Perimenopause," Magnolia writes:

Julia thank you so much for commenting and sharing your story.... I featured your post in "Dear Magnolia" today because your story is a good example of how marriages can survive perimenopause. In fact, there have been women who have reached out to me when they were going through perimenopause who shared that their husbands were extremely helpful and supportive. So, it is important to point out that if a marriage is stressed and strained during perimenopause, it is not necessarily doomed to end in divorce. Perimenopause, as I have often said, does not make a good marriage bad. It doesn't create problems in a marriage which didn't exist before. It will, however, shine a very bright light on them. Particularly if they have lingered for a very long time unresolved, shoved to the back burner of life. Those marriages which do not survive perimenopause (and I include my own in those numbers) are the marriages which were already troubled, stressed, strained, and unhealthy in the first place.... All of that said, not all women have loving, supportive husbands who help them through perimenopause. Some men simply do not know what to do—and I offer grace to those men. But others simply do not care to know, much less offer loving support. (30 Aug. 2014)

Analyses of support speak also show how a lack of supportive re-lationships affects women's talk about their perimenopausal experiences. Outside of marriage, relationships with other women, sisters, mothers or friends may be characterized as non-existent or underwhelming. Absent mothers and/or mothers who had hysterectomies are perceived to be unhelpful. Angie posts: "My mom had a full hysterectomy at age thirty, so she isn't much of a support simply because she hasn't experienced quite the same thing. What do you recommend for support as my husband simply does not understand? He tries and is very kind, but he is male. We have four teenagers, and I feel overwhelmed" (1 Jan. 2016). She-RA indicates:

I had no idea what was happening to me (my mother never shared her experiences with me, so I was taken by surprise to say the least!).... I read once we should hang on tight at this time of life; it's a crazy journey but once we get to the other side, we'll be right as rain again. I for one, am looking forward to getting out the other side.... I must be nearly there, surely! (5 Nov. 2015)

E Neilson comments:

I just turned forty.... I am dealing with weight gain, depression, anxiety, and anger.... My mom is gone, my sister does not talk to me, and, yes, doctors have told me I am too young to feel the way I am feeling. I don't know what to do—for me as much as for getting my husband to understand. If something does not give— it will surely be the end of us. Your website has been SO very helpful to me and validating that I am not crazy, nor am I too young, and that I know exactly how I am feeling.... I will continue to read.... I find it quite comforting. Thank you. (16 June 2014)

Women clearly pursue emotional support via "Dear Magnolia," which may be indicative of their struggle to find meaningful support in their face-to-face relationships. A perceived lack of emotional support not only affects relationships with spouses, family members, or friends during perimenopause but also seems to affect how they experience perimenopause. My reading of this support speak suggests Magnolia and her commenters both provide and receive emotional support. They strive to meet women's relational needs, but they tend to do so in different ways. Magnolia is mostly a "provider of support" (Inagaki and Orehek).

Still she situates herself in discussions, sharing aspects of her own story. She mentions women who have "reached out to her" or posts that have "inspired" or "touched her." My sense is connecting, listening, and empathizing with readers benefits Magnolia, too. She seems to enjoy helping, enriching her role as a support giver. Support giving may be rewarding; it affirms her capacity to bring women together. As blog author, she socially integrates perimenopausal women within her self-made supportive community. Expressions of reader gratitude nurture her sense of self and self-esteem and enhance her personal health and wellbeing. Recent research attests to my suggestion, which cites positive outcomes for support providers such as increased feelings of self-esteem and self-worth as well as more social connections (Inagaki and Orehek). In this respect, the emotional support evident in women's support speak may be understood as narratively co-constructed. It is reciprocal and of mutual benefit.

Conclusion

Women want social support during perimenopause, and they want to talk to other women going through perimenopause. *The Perimenopause Blog* is tailor made for these social interactions that perimenopausal women so desire. Women who visit "Dear Magnolia" are delighted and relieved to have found a supportive community. It helps reduce feelings of social isolation. Women are reassured that they need not go through perimenopause alone. Their feelings are normalized, and their experiences are validated. Magnolia and her readers can engage in the give and take of informational and emotional social support. "Dear Magnolia" may be read as a means by which some women's relational needs are met, especially when the existing support networks of family and friends leave much to be desired.

This supportive community encourages meaningful talk among women about perimenopause. As agentic subjects, Magnolia and readers are involved in the narrative co-construction of perimenopausal talk. Women talk about perimenopause as a transitional period in their lives. A temporary process, it reflects a passage of time marked by bodily and psychological changes. Change may also be social in nature, including changing perceptions of self or social status. Perimenopause can be difficult to endure, but transitional talk assures readers it does not last forever even if, at times, many women feel that way. Women, Magnolia included, are comforted by the talk of women who have made it to the "other side."

"Dear Magnolia" creates space for women to openly talk about perimenopausal symptoms. Symptom speak enables women to express their concerns. Navigating symptoms and treatment options can be challenging and overwhelming. These hardships are recognized. Talking about their symptoms does not magically make them go away, but engaging in such talk may make symptoms more tolerable, helping women feel better able to cope with perimenopause.

Women talk about their need for social support during perimenopause. Support speak is a two-way process. Readers post questions, search for answers, and seek support. Magnolia offers informational support, as do readers on occasion. Citing a lack of meaningful support in their existing support networks and/or relationships, Magnolia and her commenters share in the exchange of emotional support. Readers are appreciative of this support, empowering Magnolia as a support giver. This give and take is mutually beneficial.

"Dear Magnolia" embraces talk among women about perimenopause and supports women braving "the bumpy ride through perimenopause" (Miller, "About"). Granted, these narratives are largely crafted within the context of a North American English-speaking blog. Self-selected participants comprise this convenience sample. Some women may be more or less likely to blog about perimenopause. Others are perhaps content to lurk. Demographic characteristics of readers, save for perhaps age and marital status, are for the most part unknown. Data on race, social class, and sexual orientation are unavailable, raising questions related to narrative representativeness and generalizability. The anonymity, identity, and potential deception by readers may be a concern (Wilson, Kenny, and Dickson-Swift 3). That said, online anonymity may enable talk among women that differs from talk with close family or friends, allowing women to express their thoughts and feelings without fear of possible recrimination or judgment. As such, the truthfulness or authenticity of this talk and commentary is less worrisome to me. What is not being said, or the gaps or omissions in women's perimenopausal talk, may be of further sociological interest. These silences may be telling and set the stage for future study.

After spending the better part of a decade building up *The Perimeno-pause Blog*, establishing a social media presence, and dedicating countless hours engaging with loyal readers and followers, in the fall of 2018, Magnolia announced she was stepping away from her blog (7 Oct. 2018). Now several years postmenopause, she says she made the tough decision to "close up shop on the issue" and "pass the baton" on to a new team (11 Nov. 2018). While Magnolia moves on to other things and a new stage of her life, it is my hope that this chapter honours the supportive community she created to the benefit of so many women and acknowledges her blog as part of the larger historical record of how women use their relationship and community-building skills to support one another during transitional times.

Endnotes

1. Statistics Canada data from 2009 indicate roughly 70 per cent of Canadians were inclined to look up health information online, an increase from approximately 58 per cent in 2005 (Statistics Canada qtd. in Tonsaker, Bartlett, and Trpkov 407).

2. Magnolia's homepage offers a wealth of information related to symptoms of perimenopause, health and fitness, research and news items, and alternative treatments alongside the following medical disclaimer: "No information on this website is meant to be con-structed as medical advice. All content is for informational purposes only and should not be relied upon for medical diagnosis or as an alternative to medical advice from your doctor or other healthcare professional. If you are suffering from a medical condition or have any specific questions about any medical matter, consult your doctor or other professional healthcare provider" ("About The Peri-menopausal Blog").

3. For ethical reasons, it is important to note that all posts may be characterized as "open access," "nonlogin," and "nonpassword protected" (see for example Kotliar; Hookway); in other words, they are archived submissions that anyone on the internet can easily access and read.

Works Cited

Baird, D. "Negotiating the Maze: The Meaning of Perimenopause." *New Jersey Nurse*, vol. 34, no. 4, 2003, pp. 17-18.

Bresnahan, Mary Jiang, and Lisa Murray-Johnson. "The Healing Web." *Health Care for Women International*, vol. 23, no. 4, 2002, pp. 398-407.

Brown, Amy, Peter Raynor, and Michelle Lee. "Young Mothers Who Choose to Breast Feed: The Importance of Being Part of a Supportive Breast-Feeding Community." *Midwifery*, vol. 27, no. 1, 2011, pp. 53-59.

Cohen, Sheldon, Lynn G. Underwood, and Benjamin H. Gottlieb, eds. *Social Support Measurement and Intervention: A Guide for Health and Social Scientists*. Oxford University Press, 2000.

Coulson, Neil S. "Receiving Social Support Online: An Analysis of a Computer-Mediated Support Group for Individuals Living with Irritable Bowel Syndrome." *CyberPsychology & Behavior*, vol. 8, no. 6, 2005, pp. 580-84.

Coulson, Neil S., and Rebecca C. Knibb. "Coping with Food Allergy: Exploring the Role of the Online Support Group." *CyberPsychology & Behavior*, vol. 10, no. 1, 2007, pp. 145-48.

Coulson, Neil S., Heather Buchanan, and Aimee Aubeeluck. "Social Support in Cyberspace: A Content Analysis of Communication within a Huntington's Disease Online Support Group."*Patient Education and Counseling*, vol. 68, no. 2, 2007, pp. 173-78.

Cowie, Genevieve, Sophie Hill, and Priscilla Robinson. "Using an Online Service for Breastfeeding Support: What Mothers Want to Discuss." *Health Promotion Journal of Australia*, vol. 22, no. 2, 2011, pp. 113-18.

Dare, Julie, and Lelia Green. "Rethinking Social Support in Women's Midlife years: Women's Experiences of Social Support in Online Environments." *European Journal of Cultural Studies*, vol. 14, no. 5, 2011, pp. 473-90.

Dillaway, Heather E. "'Why Can't You Control This?': How Women's Interactions with Intimate Partners Define Menopause and Family." *Journal of Women & Aging*, vol. 20, no. 1-2, 2008, pp. 47-64.

Dillaway, Heather E. *Menopause in Social Context: Women's Experiences of Reproductive Aging in the United States.* 2002. Michigan State University, Unpublished PhD dissertation.

Djuraskovic, Ogi, and FirstSiteGuide Team. "What is a Blog?—The Definition of Blog, Blogging, and Blogger." *First Site Guide*, 15 Nov. 2018, firstsiteguide.com/what-is-blog/. Accessed 4 Feb. 2019.

Duffy, O. K., L. Iversen, and P. C. Hannaford. "The Impact and Management of Symptoms Experienced at Midlife: A Community Based Study of Women in Northeast Scotland." *BJOG: An International Journal of Obstetrics & Gynaecology*, vol. 119, no. 5, 2012, pp. 554-64.

Eichhorn, Kristen Campbell. "Soliciting and Providing Social Support over the Internet: An Investigation of Online Eating Disorder Support Groups." *Journal of Computer Mediated Communication*, vol. 14, no. 1, 2008, pp. 67-78.

Elder, Jessica, and Laurie A. Burke. "Parental Grief Expression in Online Cancer Support Groups." *Illness, Crisis & Loss*, vol. 23, no. 2, 2015, pp. 175-90.

Frederiksen, Eva, Janet Harris, and Karen Moland. "Web-based Discussion Forums on Pregnancy Complaints and Maternal Literacy in Norway: A Qualitative Study." *Journal of Medical Internet Research*, vol. 18, no. 5, 2016, p. e113

Gold, Katherine, Margaret Normandin, and Martha Boggs. "Are Participants in Face-to-Face and Internet Support Groups the Same? Comparison of Demographics and Depression Levels among Women Bereaved by Stillbirth." *Archives of Women's Mental Health*, vol. 19, no. 6, 2016, pp. 1073-78.

Hall, Joanne, and Jill Powell. "Understanding the Person through Narrative." *Nursing Research and Practice*. 2011;2011:293837. doi: 10.1155/2011/293837.

Hong, Yan, Ninfa C. Pena-Purcell, and Marcia G. Ory. "Outcomes of Online Support and Resources for Cancer Survivors: A Systematic Literature Review." *Patient Education and Counseling*, vol. 86, no. 3, 2012, pp. 288-96.

Hookway, Nicholas. "'Entering the Blogosphere': Some Strategies for Using Blogs in Social Research." *Qualitative Research*, vol. 8, no. 1, 2008, pp. 91-113.

Huh, Jina, et al. "Health Vlogs as Social Support for Chronic Illness Management." *ACM Transactions on Computer-Human Interaction* (TOCHI), vol. 21, no. 4, 2014, p. 23.

Hunting, Vali Sunshine. "Social Support for New Mothers: An Exploration of New Mothers' Postpartum Experiences with Online and Offline Peer Support Environments." 2009. University of Victoria, dissertation, dspace.library.uvic.ca:8443/handle/1828/1800. Accessed 18 Aug. 2020

Inagaki, Tristen K., and Edward Orehek. "On the Benefits of Giving Social Support: When, Why, and How Support Providers Gain by Caring for Others." *Current Directions in Psychological Science*, vol. 26, no. 2, 2017, pp. 109-13.

Im, Eurn-Ok et al. "A National Multiethnic Online Forum Study on Menopausal Symptom Experience." *Nursing Research*, vol. 59, no. 1, 2010, pp. 26-33.

Johnson, Sophia Alice. "'Intimate Mothering Publics': Comparing Face-to-Face Support Groups and Internet Use for Women Seeking Information and Advice in the Transition to First-Time Motherhood." *Culture, Health & Sexuality*, vol. 17, no. 2, 2015, pp. 237-51.

Ko, Hsiu-Chia, Li-Ling Wang, and Yi-Ting Xu. "Understanding the Different Types of Social Support Offered by Audience to A-List Diary-Like and Informative Bloggers." *Cyberpsychology, Behavior, and Social Networking*, vol. 16, no. 3, 2013, pp. 194-99.

Koch, Patricia Barthalow, and Phyllis Kernoff Mansfield. "Facing the Unknown: Social Support during the Menopausal Transition." *Women & Therapy*, vol. 27, no. 3-4, 2004, pp. 179-94.

Kotliar, Dan M. "Depression Narratives in Blogs: A Collaborative Quest for Coherence." *Qualitative Health Research*, vol. 26, no. 9, 2016, pp. 1203-15.

Letourneau, Nicole, et al. "Impact of Online Support for Youth with Asthma and Allergies: Pilot Study." *Journal of Pediatric Nursing*, vol. 27, no. 1, 2012, pp. 65-73.

Ley, Barbara. "Vive les Roses!: The Architecture of Commitment in an Online Pregnancy and Mothering Group." *Journal of Computer-Mediated Communication*, vol. 12, no. 4, 2007, pp. 1388-1408.

Mansfield, Phyllis Kernoff, Patricia Barthalow Koch, and Gretchen Gierach. "Husbands' Support of Their Perimenopausal Wives." *Women & Health*, vol. 38, no. 3, 2003, pp. 97-112.

Mattson, Marifran, and Jennifer Gibb Hall. *Health as Communication Nexus: A Service-Learning Approach*. Kendal Hunt, 2011.

Miller, Magnolia. "About The Perimenopausal Blog." *The Perimenopausal Blog*, Pink Zinnia, 5 Feb. 2019. www.theperimenopauseblog.com/about-the-perimenopause-blog/. Accessed 10 Mar. 2021.

Miller, Magnolia. "Archives." *The Perimenopause Blog*. Pink Zinnia. 10 Feb. 2017, www.theperimenopauseblog.com/category/dear-magnolia. Accessed 10 Mar. 2021.

Miller, Magnolia. "My (Hormone-Filled and Bumpy) Ride Through Perimenopause." *Ageology*, 20 Sept. 2013, www.ageology.com/my-hormone-filled-and-bumpy-ride-through-perimenopause/. Accessed 27 Feb. 2019.

Nolan, Samantha et al. "Social Networking Site (SNS) Use by Adolescent Mothers": Can Social Support and Social Capital Be Enhanced by Online Social Networks?—A Structured Review of the Literature." *Midwifery*, vol. 48, 2017, pp. 24-31.

Orgad, Shani. *Storytelling Online: Talking Breast Cancer on the Internet*. Peter Lang, 2005.

Pedersen, Sarah, and Caroline Macafee. "Gender Differences in British Blogging." *Journal of Computer Mediated Communication*, vol. 12, no. 4, 2007, pp. 1472-92.

Rains, Stephen A., and David M. Keating. "The Social Dimension of Blogging about Health: Health Blogging, Social Support, and Well-Being." *Communication Monographs*, vol. 78, no. 4, 2011, pp. 511-34.

Reece, Susan M. and Gene E. Harkless. "Perimenopausal Health Self-Efficacy among Hispanic Caribbean and Non-Hispanic White Women." *Health Care for Women International*, vol. 7, no. 3, 2006, pp. 223-37.

Seale, Clive. "Gender Accommodation in Online Cancer Support Groups." *Health*, vol. 10, no. 3, 2006, pp. 345-60.

Seale, Clive, Sue Ziebland, and Jonathan Charteris-Black. "Gender, Cancer Experience and Internet Use: A Comparative Keyword

Analysis of Interviews and Online Cancer Support Groups." *Social Science & Medicine*, vol. 62, no. 10, 2006, pp. 2577-90.

Sillence, Elizabeth, et al. "How do patients evaluate and make use of online health information?" *Social Science & Medicine*, vol. 64, no. 9, 2007, pp. 1853-62.

Sosnowy, Collette. *Blogging Chronic Illness and Negotiating Patient-Hood: Online Narratives of Women with MS*. City University of New York, 2013.

Soules, Michael R., et al. "Executive Summary: Stages of Reproductive Aging Workshop (STRAW) Park City, Utah, July, 2001." *Menopause*, vol. 8, no. 6, 2001, pp. 402-07.

Statistics Canada. "Internet Use by Individuals, by Type of Activity (Internet Users at Home) Statistics Canada, CANSIM, table 358-0130. Last modified: 2010-05-10." Statistics Canada, 2010, www.statcan.gc.ca/tables-tableaux/sum-som/l01/cst01/comm29a-eng.htm. Accessed 8 Mar. 2016.

Teaford, Dominique, Deepika Goyal, and Susan McNiesh. "Identification of Postpartum Depression in an Online Community." *Journal of Obstetric Gynecologic and Neonatal Nursing*, vol. 55, no. 5, 2015, pp. 578-86.

Thompson, Jennifer Jo. *Managing Menopause: An Ethnographic Study of Women's Midlife Information-Seeking and Decision-Making in the Southwest US*. 2010. University of Georgia, PhD dissertation.

Tonsaker, Tabitha, Gillian Bartlett, and Cvetan Trpkov. "Health Information on the Internet: Gold Mine or Minefield?" *Canadian Family Physician*, vol. 60, no. 5, 2014, pp. 407-08.

Trudeau, Kimberlee J., et al. "Identifying the Educational Needs of Menopausal Women: A Feasibility Study." *Women's Health Issues*, vol. 21, no. 2, 2011, pp. 145-52.

Turner, Jacob S. "Negotiating a Media Effects Model: Addendums and Adjustments to Perloff's Framework for Social Media's Impact on Body Image Concerns." *Sex Roles*, vol. 71, no. 11-12, 2014, pp. 393-406.

Vilhauer, Ruvanee P. "Perceived Benefits of Online Support Groups for Women with Metastatic Breast Cancer." *Women & Health*, vol. 49, no. 5, 2009, pp. 381-404.

Weinert, Clarann. "Social Support in Cyberspace for Women with Chronic Illness." *Rehabilitation Nursing*, vol. 25, no. 4, 2000, pp. 129-35.

Weinert, Clarann, Shirley Cudney, and Charlene Winters. "Social Support in Cyberspace: The Next Generation." *Computers, Informatics, Nursing*, vol. 23, no. 1, 2005, pp. 7-15.

White, Marsha, and Steve M. Dorman. "Receiving Social Support Online: Implications for Health Education." *Health Education Research*, vol. 16, no. 6, 2001, pp. 693-707.

Wilson, Elena, Amanda Kenny, and Virginia Dickson-Swift. "Using Blogs as a Qualitative Health Research Tool: A Scoping Review." *International Journal of Qualitative Methods*, vol. 14, no. 5, 2015, https://doi.org/10.1177/1609406915618049.

Chapter 12

Finding Bedrock

Marie Maccagno

As a forty-something woman, I blithely imagined I would sail through perimenopause to menopause without the myriad of symptoms I'd heard and read about. One of my writing mentors uses an exercise that starts with the sentence stem: "Tell me everything you know about _____." If I had filled in the blank with "menopause" prior to my lived experience, I would have written something like this:

> Menopause is overblown in our culture. I've been looking after my body well, and my alternative medical support has been proactive, preparing my body for the changes coming soon, I'm not likely to have many symptoms. I believe that menopause is a myth the allopathic medical system has made up to medicalize a natural female process. It's just another way for the capitalist system to profit from drugs to administer, organs to cut out, and emotions to dismiss because of women's hormones.

Now, looking back twelve years after reaching menopause, what I would write is "This shit is real!" The experience was not just about the physical changes, the weight gain, mood swings, and hot flashes. Exploring questions about gender definitions and life purpose as a woman no longer able to bear children, along with deep-seated creative desires clamouring for attention, required intense emotional labour. From my sixty-something perspective, I now realize the revolution I experienced went far beyond hot flashes and dry vaginas. For me, perimenopause triggered the renovation of personal relationships and dramatically changed how I chose to be a partner in my marriage and mother to my now-adult children. Most profound was how it transformed my relationship with myself.

In the couple of years prior to full menopause, I resolved to fulfill a dream: to walk the Camino de Santiago in Northern Spain. My husband, Rod, and adult son would accompany me. As I prepared for our Camino pilgrimage, I was also in the midst of examining my relationship with my husband, wondering about the future of my marriage. During my Camino journey, I had many opportunities for self-reflection, the long hours of putting one foot in front of another leading to deep meditative states. Upon my return to Canada, I committed to my long-simmering desire to write. As my words flowed onto the pages, I realized I was crafting a memoir about my Camino journey. Important themes emerged that had been unleashed by the walk. I proceeded one sentence, one paragraph, one page at a time until I had a finished manuscript based on our day-to-day journey. The publication of my memoir, *The Chocolate Pilgrim: A Journey to Self-discovery and Transformation on the Camino de Santiago,* was a culmination of resolution, healing, and self-confidence.

From reading I have done since those unsettled years of questioning my self-identity and personal relationships, I've discovered that I was responding to a call that many women answer during this major transition: an invitation to live more truthfully, aligned with our innermost impulses, beliefs, and desires. Christiane Northrup writes about this call to action in *The Wisdom of Menopause:* "The primary relationship that needs updating at midlife is the one you have with yourself. All other interpersonal crises that arise at this time are simply reflections of this. What's really going on is that the new self you're becoming is no longer willing to accept less than she deserves or is capable of receiving from others." (3)

As I navigated the turbulent perimenopausal years before setting out on the Camino de Santiago, the one constant that anchored me in a state of wellbeing was the natural world. I found solace hiking the trails of the Rocky Mountains near Calgary, where I raised my children and built a psychotherapy practice, and was inspired by the coastal environment on Vancouver Island, where I moved with my husband in our early fifties. Without access to these places of beauty and wonder, I'm not sure I'd still be here to write this story.

My relationship with natural spaces began when I was a child. Although my biological mother was often harsh and unforgiving within our home, her energy shifted to curiosity and delight when we left the boundaries of our town. Some of my fondest childhood memories are adventures with Mom, whether it was fishing on a pristine river, spending a weekend at our cottage, or exploring a nearby forest. Her presence was softer in these settings, and I also found acceptance and gentleness in the forests around me.

The rural area we lived in provided plenty of access to the gentle mothering offered by trees, moss, lakes, and the mystery of our natural surroundings. Although I did not trust other humans to listen to me, when I entered a forest, I felt as if I were returning to familiar friends. I came to recognize that each season had a different scent. The fresh sap of spring, as leaves were just beginning to emerge after winter, was tangy in my nostrils. The essence of fall as the leaves dropped had the scent of decay in the air. The old trees were always good listeners. Sometimes they spoke back to me with wisdom and compassion. They stood tall and strong in their tree-ness with no judgment. Time dropped away, and I felt safe enough to enter the present moment. I could feel tension leave my shoulders, running down the back of my legs and out into the ground below. My breathing slowed, and each breath was deeper than the last. My entire body relaxed into a sense of peace, held by the loving support of the living beings around me.

At the time both of our children were preparing to leave our home, I was in the midst of "the change." In a WTF! moment, my husband also disclosed that he had been diagnosed with chronic lymphocytic leukemia (CLL). This was not part of any plans we might have had for our future, and my emotional response was strong: I felt abandoned, scared, and angry. I envisioned worst-case scenarios. It had taken Rod some time to digest his diagnosis. Even though CLL can take many years to develop to the point of requiring treatment, he felt a sense of urgency to make changes, to plan for retirement. Over the several weeks between receiving his diagnosis and disclosing to me, he started planning a move away from the booming city we lived in. I wasn't feeling ready to leave the life I'd built over more than two decades. Calgary, he insisted, was no longer a healthy place for him to live. Although we had talked about a future move, looking west to British Columbia, I was thinking several years down the road. Rod was confident he could find work as an archaeologist on the West Coast and wasn't prepared to wait much longer. Our ideal location was Vancouver Island, although it seemed like living there could only be a distant dream.

A number of unexpected circumstances brought the dream to reality. Because of the housing boom in Calgary at the time, the value of our house would allow us to purchase a home on the West Coast without requiring a mortgage. Friends told us about a cohousing community forming on Vancouver Island, so we travelled there to attend an open house. After a weekend of meeting people who could be our neighbours as well as touring the property and the area where we'd be living, we said a wholehearted "Yes" to relocating there. In addition to the opportunity of sharing a nine-acre urban property with other like-minded households, we were especially attracted to all the outdoor recreation opportunities the area provided: hiking and sea kayaking over three seasons, skiing and snowshoeing in winter, and urban walking year round through many accessible trails. Each destination we visited on that first fact-finding mission offered breathtaking beauty, with the promise in their place names of more to come: Nymph Falls, Seal Bay Park, Paradise Meadows.

I agreed to this new adventure with the belief we wouldn't be moving for at least another five years. I wanted more time for our children to settle into life on their own with their parents still nearby. I wanted more time to grow my counselling practice, to continue developing my musical interests, playing trombone in an adult concert band, and learning conversational Spanish. I hated the thought of no longer having access to my favourite yoga studio and I wasn't yet prepared to leave behind the Rocky Mountains, with all the beloved terrain I explored in winter, spring, summer, and fall.

Rather than a reprieve of five years, our new cohousing community home was ready for move-in within two years. GULP! At the same time, Rod's application to transfer his work as an archaeologist with Parks Canada to the West Coast was approved. I wasn't ready to move, but my husband was. How could I say no to a man with a possibly abbreviated life? So in 2007, I made the hard decision to leave our young adult children in Calgary and move to a new city in a new province, a thirteen-hour car and ferry journey away. Throughout the time of packing, sorting, and letting go, I was in a period of deep self-reflection. As I wrote in my memoir, even before the move:

> I began to question who I was as a woman and a wife. I reviewed
> the roles that [my husband] and I had adopted in our marriage

and wondered if I wanted to keep living in those gender-defined boxes. This was a surprise to me because the earlier version of me had been so determined to avoid repeating anything that resembled my parents' marriage. Even though Rod contributed a great deal to household chores and was a very involved parent, there were still ways we automatically defaulted to standard cultural prescriptions. Decisions about childcare? Marie's department.... Problems with kids at school? Marie's responsibility. Our daughter Emma needing emotional support? Definitely Mom's time to step up. Given our busy lives and many commitments, role definitions allowed us to function efficiently. (9)

My deep self-examination continued throughout the settling-in process. We had moved to a small city where we didn't know anyone well. Living in our new home without our children highlighted how little emotional connection I felt with my husband. I longed for the structure provided by my private practice as well as the strong network of friends and colleagues I had built up over twenty-five years of living in the same place:

> In our new home on Vancouver Island, I missed having [my children] living with us. I'd heard about the "empty nest" feeling, but I never expected that it would apply to me. Uprooting from Calgary, where I had lived for twenty-eight years, prompted me to reevaluate everything about my life. What kind of work did I want to do? What groups did I want to join? Who was I now that my children were launched? Did I want to be a wife anymore? How long did Rod have left to live? What will it be like to be left here a widow, when I don't know anyone? The effects of leaving my Calgary network of friends and work colleagues were hitting harder than I ever could have imagined. (IV)

Without the support of familiar friends and surroundings, and little sense of purpose in my life, my sense of wellbeing dissipated. I'd been prone to depression at earlier times in my life, and now I was in freefall: "My body is going through menopause, and my interest in life is swirling clockwise down a dark hole. I feel as if I have no reason to live anymore, and I can feel my senses shutting down. I don't know how to reach out.

I don't know anyone in this new community well enough to confide in. I retreat deeper into silence every day" (87-88).

For many weeks, I felt as if I were living behind plexiglass, a see-through barrier keeping me apart from the life going on around me. My nerve endings felt numb, my thought processes like thick mud sliding slowly down a shallow slope. Questions about my future circled endlessly in my brain. Now that I had raised my children, wasn't my work done? Was there any value to my life going forwards? Dark thoughts shadowed every day, and I sank into a wordless place, distant from everyone. I stopped speaking for almost fifteen weeks, unable to emerge from the prison of my despair.

Looking back, the metaphor that comes to mind is travelling through a birth canal, shedding everything that no longer served me and that had nothing to do with who I was becoming. During this transition, I was a stranger to myself. The one place I felt accepted and nourished was on the nearby forest trails. My distant dream of walking the Camino de Santiago often appeared on the periphery of my consciousness—at times vivid and at others, remote and unattainable. I spent hours walking and exploring new areas with my cohousing neighbours and one hiking group I had joined; this was how I began creating new relationships. Movement, walking, and putting one foot in front of the other unlocked my voice, although I did not disclose the depths of my despair to anyone. That felt too shameful to share.

Although I'd expected some physical changes with the hormonal fluctuations of perimenopause—the weight gain, change in muscle tone, the occasional memory scramble—I wasn't prepared for the assault on my mental health. I'd been depressed before but never anything like this. As much as I tried to push unwelcome thoughts away, they continued to bombard my senses. No matter how many techniques I tried, the relentless negative messages continued to erode my confidence and self-worth. I suspect our physical relocation exacerbated my difficulties. I walked incessantly for relief, the only hours in each day the endless squeaking hamster wheel of thoughts in my head fell silent. My inner voices kept telling me that all I was doing was occupying space; I was a burden to everyone. I truly wondered whether it was worth living, looking for ways to end my life that would look like an accident.

No matter how hard I tried, I couldn't find any reason to continue living. Parenting and income earning—two occupations that had given me a sense of self-worth and value—were gone. Without children to care for, without their needs being the primary glue of Rod's and my well-functioning, focused-on-tasks marriage, it seemed as if there was nothing left to keep us together. It was hard to admit, even to myself, that I was deeply affected by Rod's leukemia diagnosis and the possibility that I would be left on my own. His doctor had said, "Now we watch and wait." Although there were no observable physical changes at this early stage, my trust in Rod always being there for me had been shaken to the core. Without an independent source of income, my sense of freedom and ability to choose was curtailed. More often than not, I felt trapped by circumstances beyond my control, with no way out.

If our marriage was to survive, my husband and I needed to create new ways of connecting, and for almost a year, we had very few. Our connection was initially forged through outdoor activities, which continued throughout the time we raised our family. Spending time outside was one of the few bonds we continued to share on Vancouver Island. However, since Rod was away for long stretches, working on his final fieldwork season prior to retirement, my depression deepened. I had no work and was not sure what I wanted to do next. Since I was no longer earning money, I felt worthless; I discovered that my sense of value was connected to income. Before I could thrive in my new environment, old beliefs such as this had to die.

This can be a familiar experience for women in Western culture transitioning to menopause, where one common belief is that once we're no longer able to bear children, our work is done. Finding meaning in life after our reproductive ability has passed is a large part of our developmental work. On the other side of the bleeding time are opportunities to explore creative pursuits and to move beyond the confines of parenting, family, and the role of nurturing others. It's our time to develop long-simmering passions—a time for saying "yes" to what we as women most strongly desire.

I finally felt my interest in life returning at the end of summer 2008. The tidal wave of negative thinking receded as I started issuing invitations to friends, enjoying a hike with Rod, and occasionally laughing out loud. My appetite for food, which had almost completely disappeared, returned, so restaurant meals became a special treat. Rod and I were cautious with each other, since my long period of silence and withdrawal had left both of us feeling uncertain about our next steps. Would we stay together or not? This was an unspoken question between us.

Coincidentally, I had an unexpected job offer to work on a contract for a company based in Calgary. I immediately accepted and flew out on a one-way ticket. At that time, I wasn't sure if and when I'd return. That short-term contract would turn into ten years of employment in the field of environmental assessment, work that I loved. It was the beginning of a steady workload and substantial salary that gave me a sense of financial independence and freedom of movement I'd never experienced before.

Getting settled into my new job signalled the perfect time to plan our pilgrimage walk across Northern Spain. In early 2009, Rod and I, despite all the uncertainty between us, made two major decisions. The first was to buy our plane tickets to Europe; we would leave Canada in early April. The second was buying a condo in Calgary, since I needed to spend half my time in that city to complete work commitments. This purchase provided our son with stable accommodation, who moved in with two of his friends. I made a declaration to everyone that I was no one's mother, and I was not looking after any of them. "Consider me just another tenant," I said. Later, our daughter joined us when she left a long-term relationship. The condo gave her a safe place to land and begin rebuilding her life. I had to step back from my expectations for her life choices and let her craft her own path. I did my best to withhold advice or comments to either child unless I was specifically asked for suggestions. More than anything, I wanted our children to know that I would support them through both their challenges and their good times. I knew that no matter what, Rod felt the same way. We had made the shift to seeing our children as adults capable of making good decisions, even if we didn't always agree with their choices.

After returning home from our Camino adventure, I chose to pursue another life-long dream: writing a book. I now had the income to afford a year-long program combining yoga and writing—Language of Yoga—without any negative impact on my ability to pay regular or unexpected expenses. I kept it a secret from my husband.

Because the program was based in Calgary and I was spending at least half my time in that city, it was easy not to mention it to Rod. I structured my work and travel schedule to coincide with weekend writing workshops and one-on-one coaching sessions. While I was travelling back and forth between Calgary and Vancouver Island, he was making good use of his solo time. The CLL was still progressing slowly, and his health was robust. I felt comfortable being away because I knew he was well supported by all our neighbours. He also had a major project to focus on while I was away: completing his PhD thesis. Whenever I returned home, I didn't yet feel ready to share my new commitment to writing. Any suggestion of "that's a bad idea," or "you shouldn't spend all that money" could have shaken my commitment.

I finally told Rod about the program when I chose to reenroll for a second year. He was upset, wondering why I didn't trust him enough to tell him when I first joined the Language of Yoga. I'm not sure how much lack of trust was involved, but I do know why I didn't tell him. Although Rod had done his best to be supportive of my decisions throughout our relationship, his support was often couched in the energy of devil's advocate. His academic training would kick in, compelling him to make sure that I had considered all the possible ways I might fail, as well as the benefits. I could easily imagine being peppered with questions and statements like "Are you sure you really want to do that?" "That's a lot of money" and "Aren't you a little old to start writing?" Comments like these, though well intentioned, had stopped me from moving forwards before. So I chose silence as my strategy until I was stronger in my conviction.

Following my deepest desires, without concern for what other people thought, was a newly germinating seed in my life, not a well-established practice. Up until now, I had excelled at being a "pleaser." My desire to belong and to be liked meant that I hadn't always chosen what I truly wanted; instead, I did what I thought others wanted me to do. But during this menopausal shift, I started to notice how much time I spent wondering what other people might want me to do. I noticed that I often imagined what people were thinking about me and worried about doing the wrong thing. I'd review a series of events, questioning whether I should have done X, Y, or Z differently. I eventually resolved to stop this pattern.

Time in the forests around me was a great teacher. After moving to Vancouver Island, I became less focused on destination hiking and more content to saunter in the woods, mindfully observing all the living beings around me. This was a big shift from the hiking I had done in the Rockies, where I often pushed myself to cover great distances. With this new approach, I discovered it was helpful to ask myself what nonhuman forms might have to say about how I behaved. As crazy as it may sound, I would find myself checking in with a wise Douglas fir or a compassionate cedar. I felt the trees affirming my decision to wait before disclosing my commitment to writing.

The lessons from nature extended to all aspects of my life. Observing the differences between my mind state and the elements in nature taught me that my potential creative energy was often diverted into anxiety and worry, questioning and self-doubt. I learned that I could draw on the properties of the natural world to support me when I was emotionally volatile. If I was having a particularly neurotic day, I discovered I could connect with the properties of bedrock exposed in the higher elevations of Vancouver Island. I experienced this geological formation as supremely confident, beyond self-doubt and reproach. When I embodied the qualities of bedrock by standing firm in my core beliefs, I could harness and direct my creative power.

My decision to pursue writing ended up benefitting our whole family. I eventually completed my memoir and launched my book in the fall of 2017. In order to follow through on my dreams—whether it was walking the Camino or publishing my book—I had to continue believing in what was possible. I was no longer content staying within my previous comfort zone, relying on what was safe and predictable. Whatever lessons I learned about nurturing creativity, responding to crappy first drafts, and honouring every step of the way have been transmitted to our children. My husband gradually gave himself permission to pursue his creative goals as well, taking classes and eventually becoming a ceramic artist. I've modelled the process rather than lectured. I've learned we can change our relationship dynamics by showing up differently, and my life is proof of that. When I stopped making myself small to make my husband comfortable, everything changed between us.

Whereas many older women describe feeling invisible at midlife and beyond, I don't. In order to support the sales of my memoir, I started public speaking. I was so passionate about the transformation that's possible through writing I established a business as a writing mentor and guide. I never would have envisioned this version of Marie during my forties. As a child, and throughout my early adult years, I often felt invisible to people around me, perhaps because I so seldom spoke from the truth inside of me. I tended to adapt to the opinions and beliefs of whatever group I was in so I wouldn't stand out in any way. Being singled out meant danger; I chose safety in conforming. Now I can choose when to step back into the shadows and when to stand in the spotlight.

One of the most valuable aspects of my time in the year-long writing program was sharing my experience with other participants who were all on a path of self-development. All through our time together we worked on our growth—reflecting back each other's strengths, noticing where we had blind spots, holding each other in our vulnerabilities. The group experience, perhaps more than any other, helped me to move beyond my long-held sense of being invisible. I discovered there is nothing more painful than being unaware of my deepest desires and silencing myself in order to feel safe.

In the life I am living today, I no longer make decisions according to my old childhood criteria. I share my hopes and dreams with my husband, who thankfully has survived several rounds of treatment for his illness and continues to thrive. We now know how to fully support each other. We continue to savour our relationships with our children and their partners, feeling blessed with all the ways we share time and laughter together. As we have each learned to say "yes" to our individual desires, we also connect more deeply as a family. I am grateful for all the questioning I did during those perimenopausal years, for the painful challenges I surmounted, and for the unexpected twists and turns of discovery that guided me to the bedrock I now stand upon.

Works Cited

Maccagno, Marie. *The Chocolate Pilgrim: A Journey of Self-discovery & Transformation on the Camino de Santiago.* Adventures in Writing, 2017.

Northrup, Christiane. "Relationships." *The Wisdom of Menopause Journal.* Hay House USA, 2007.

Chapter 13

Menopause Claimed

Laura Wershler

We sat in a circle around a makeshift altar, small and low to the ground, covered with a crimson cloth embossed with long-stemmed flowers upon which lay a speckled stone beside a tuft of animal fur, white sage and a shallow round shell to catch its ashes, a burning white candle in a red transparent holder, and a piece of pale yellow-white coral. Each object, we were told, was placed in reference to the four directions and represented one of the four elements—earth, air, fire, water. The tightly rolled ball of red yarn in the centre symbolized our bloodlines and our interrelatedness. The ritual was about to begin.

Rites of Passage: Reclaiming Women's Rites—a workshop scheduled on the last day of the 2015 biennial conference of the Society for Menstrual Cycle Research in Boston, Massachusetts—had attracted close to twenty women of varying ages and fields of menstrual endeavour. After two days of intense exploration into research, advocacy, and artistic perspectives on the central role the menstrual cycle plays in women's health and lives, I was ready for a more personal experience. According to the conference program, the workshop proposed to identify key rites of passage and "gain a new perspective on the potential for ritual and ceremony—outside of a religious context—to support health and wellbeing."

Ceremonialist Giuliana Serena began by inviting us to introduce ourselves and share what brought us to the conference and to this session. She asked us to be "lean with our words," an instruction each woman followed with carefully focused statements. As the circle of introductions came to a close, I confirmed that I was the oldest participant by several years, possibly the only one who had aged out and ceased to bleed by natural cause.

Menopause had occurred for me eight years before at fifty-four, the age at which I had gone one year without a day of bleeding. My perimenopausal transition had been a relatively smooth one. No heavy bleeding. No sleep-depriving night sweats. No weight gain. No sense of loss as my fertility waned. I had charted my signs of fertility from age twenty-seven on, at first using only my Day-Timer calendar to mark days with cervical mucus (which denoted my fertile phase) and the day on which I felt the unmistakable and sometimes searing pain of ovulation. (On that space in the calendar, I wrote R or L—to designate the side on which I felt the twenty-four hour ache of an egg breaking through my ovary—surrounded by an O.) I ovulated consistently throughout my late twenties, thirties, and forties, and I effectively used self-taught fertility awareness as birth control throughout that time, having one pregnancy, intended, when I was thirty.

At forty-eight, I began to keep more formal records using paper charts, designed for women practicing fertility awareness, to record my observations of menstrual flow, cervical mucus, basal body temperature, and variables related to exercise, illness, stress, travel, and other miscellaneous details. I expected to document the onset of cyclic changes and problematic perimenopausal symptoms I had read about, but little changed for me. My cycles shortened from around thirty-two to twenty-six or twenty-seven days, but I was still ovulating regularly. My charts told me that my luteal phases—number of days from ovulation to first day of next period—were also shorter, signalling my reduced chance of becoming pregnant. I experienced sleep disturbances, waking at four in the morning and not getting back to sleep. In my mid- to late-forties, my normal cyclic mood swings intensified. I described this in an article I wrote in 2006: "Instead of feeling blue, I felt depressed. Instead of feeling cheerful, I felt manic." Charting gave me the power to both expect these feelings and know they would pass. As I also noted, "My cycle had been a touchstone for both my sexual and reproductive health and my overall well-being." This personal experience of connection to my body had motivated my work in menstrual cycle advocacy and body literacy[1] as well as my involvement with the Society for Menstrual Cycle Research.

With introductions completed, Giuliana began a guided visualization through the "blood rites," inviting us to feel deeply into our memories of menarche and menstruation, sexuality, pregnancy and birth, miscarriage or abortion or other loss, and menopause. If we'd not experienced key rites of passage ourselves, we were to think about women we knew who had: our friends, sisters, aunts, mothers, grandmothers. What gave us the most charge? Which experience or memory caught and held fast in our consciousness? "Hang on to that," Giuliana said. Oddly, what stuck in my mind was the recent loss of my mother who had passed away three months short of her ninety-sixth birthday, just over a year before. She died slowly of old age over a three-year span during which she lived in a long-term care community fifteen minutes from my home. I was still recovering from the physical and emotional exhaustion of being her primary family care provider, of watching my beloved mother struggle with advancing frailty. I realized at that moment that only when she was gone, when I was sixty years old, did I feel as if I had finally reached menopause.

Before I could delve more deeply into this revelation, we were standing in front of large pieces of flip-chart paper taped to the walls and were asked to write down our memories under the same rites-of-passage headings that had guided the visualization. Most of my memories had some connection to my mother. I remembered the note I left on her dresser when I was twelve or thirteen with a simple question: "Will you take me to the store to buy a bra?" Below the question, I'd drawn two small boxes beside the words "yes" and "no." She checked the "yes" box and returned the note to my dresser top. As a public health nurse, she had prepared me well for the onset of my period—giving me a booklet to read she'd brought home from work, making herself available for conversation, modelling comfort. I remembered sitting on the open stairway in our split-level home, asking her questions as she made dinner in the kitchen, my father and two older brothers conveniently absent. When my period came, I told her without hesitation or embarrassment, and she brought me the belt and pads she had stored away ready and waiting.

I remembered my horribly painful cramps, the missed days of school spent in bed, twisting and turning in agony, waiting for the spasms to end and sleep to come. My mother nursed me with hot water bottles and painkillers, offered solace and sympathy. She took me to our family doctor who took my pain seriously, perhaps, I realize now, only because of my mother's insistence. In 1968, I surely was one of the first Canadian teenagers prescribed the birth control pill for off-label use—to manage dysmenorrhea. When the pill didn't alleviate my pain, our doctor wrote a prescription for anti-inflammatory medication. Over the years, I learned other ways to minimize my painful periods—avoid sugar, give myself orgasms. When I began charting my cycles and knew when to expect my period, I took ibuprofen before the bleeding started, which was the most effective method I found to prevent the grip of debilitating cramps. As my body literacy grew, my relationship with my body flourished. It became known to me, understood, appreciated.

These memories, refracted through the prism of ritual to reveal previously hidden significance, prompted me to wonder: Can I trace my life-long commitment to women's sexual and reproductive health back to my mother's practical and respectful responses to my experiences of menarche and menstruation? Is she the reason I never hated my period and, ultimately, became a menstrual cycle advocate?

I paused before the sheet headed "Miscarriage/Abortion/Loss," thinking about my cousin who had lost a baby, born prematurely at seven months with a heart defect, a boy who would have grown up with my son, born one month later. My birth-experience memory brought me back to my mother. My son was born two weeks early, at half-past twelve noon on a hot July day in 1984. I'd gone into labour at three in the morning, not the time to alert anyone. In the hours after his birth, my husband called our family and friends to share our happy news. But he could not find my parents. By the time he reached where they were staying on a visit to relatives in another province, they had left for home. Thinking they might make the nine-hour drive in one day, I called their house several times that evening from the hospital pay phone. There was no answer. After I breastfed my son, the night nurse, finding my blood pressure to be high, scolded me into bed, telling me to get some rest. As I tried to settle into sleep, my fatigue melted into an aching sadness, a deep need for my parents to know I'd had my baby. My enormous love for him could not be contained by my heart alone; it needed my mother's heart to spill into. I was in awe of this love, and when it struck me that this is what my mother must have felt for me, a pure, tingling, orgasmic sensation flushed slowly through my body from head to toes. This was her love washing through me, enveloping me, as if it had been floating in the atmosphere for thirty years waiting for me to discover it. Forty-eight hours after my son was born, when my mother was holding him for the first time, only then, it seemed to me, had he fully entered this world.

As I moved from paper sheet to paper sheet, I added phrases and sentences that summarized my rites of passage. Reading other women's words had me wondering if they, too, were reliving similarly intense experiences, finding new insights in old memories. The room was silent save for the rustling of bodies in motion, the soft squeak of felt pens on paper, but it bristled with currents of energy that prickled my skin. When we returned to our chairs in the circle, Giuliana brought us back to focus by explaining what came next. In groups of three, we were asked to share the experience that had resonated most deeply. I knew and admired the other women in my small group, having met them both at the same conference two years previously. Familiarity with one another's work and the safe space created by our facilitator urged us forwards. These two young women, decades younger than I, shared experiences tinged with regret, familial love, inspiration, sadness, eroticism, discovery, wrapped in stories that are only theirs to tell. I shared what I had realized just that day—that only when my mother died, did I feel as if I had finally reached menopause.

It was odd, I told them, how the physical and emotional strain of caring for my mother over the many months she lived in long-term care surfaced cyclically to overwhelm me. Every three months or so, fatigue and sorrow forged into heart-pounding anxiety that unleashed tears and rage at everyone and everything. During those periods, I sometimes had to force myself to get in the car and drive fifteen minutes to see my mother. I wondered at the cyclicality of these meltdowns. Was it because I was menopausal that they were seasonal and not monthly? Yet they seemed to serve the same purpose as those premenstrual windows of clarity through which I had seen exactly what mattered to me the most, bothered me the most, challenged most my imagination of self. Between these bouts of dysphoria, I often agonized over my lack of personal productivity, worried that I was using my mother as an excuse to avoid my own present, perhaps even my future. Who was I? Who was I supposed to be? Who might I be under different circumstances? I resented my confusion. I handled this resentment like a hot potato, tossing it back and forth between different versions of myself with little resolve. But while caught in these cyclic hurricanes of swirling anger and grief, I'd realize that who I wanted to be, who I needed to be, who I could only be during this time was the daughter and companion of an elderly woman whose life was slowly drawing to a close. I could not ignore that I was in the midst of the transition that would leave me motherless. I chose presence over distraction. Resentment gave way to compassion—for myself and my mother. Only when she died, did my sense of living cyclically dissolve.

Soft murmuring from the other small groups drew to a close when Giuliana asked us to finish our discussions and rejoin the circle. We three hugged and wiped away a few tears. I felt cracked open to the emotional energy coursing through the room, but at the same time relaxed and placid, as if every muscle in my body had softened around my bones. We took our places around the small altar, where the white candle still burned. One woman from each group reported on the themes of the stories we had shared in our threesomes. Then, our final step in the day's ritual began. At Giuliani's invitation, mindful of her repeated guidance to "be lean with our words," we went around the circle once again, in turn saying our names, what we were feeling, and what we would take away to celebrate. In each woman's concise declaration, our visualizations through the blood rites, our reclaimed memories, apprehended insights, and shared stories transformed into ceremonial observances rich with meaning. As each took her turn to speak, energy diffused into the circle, vibrating with the tension of competing perceptions: exasperation and inspiration, frustration and liberation, mutilation and wholeness, pain and the relief of pain, sadness and joy. Emotions lost and emotions found.

My placement in the circle meant that my turn would come close to last. As woman after woman spoke, I began to sense something swelling inside me, rising upwards towards my heart. Their words and feelings were filling me slowly but inexorably. I was an open vessel, incapable of closing myself off to the alchemical power wrought by the ritual we had shared. What they felt, I felt; what they feared, I feared; what they hoped for, I hoped for; what they forgave, I forgave. Their gratitude became my gratitude. Closer and closer, my turn was coming. The swelling inside of me rose to reach my throat. I could barely swallow; I doubted I could speak. Tears began to flow down my face. Were they mine alone or was I crying for all of us? I sat still, head up, face forwards, receiving what now seemed like offerings from the hearts of these women.

When it was my turn to speak my eyes were still streaming, but I was not sobbing. All I could say was "I'm not sure what's happening." I could see concern on some of their faces, bewilderment on others. I, too, was bewildered. Those beside me gently patted my back, offered me tissues. "I don't even know why I'm crying," I said. Whatever else I might have said is lost to my memory, consumed by the enormity of the experience. My body was responding instinctively without my conscious understanding of how or why. I was at once overwhelmed and perfectly at ease. The few remaining women took their turns to speak; then, Giuliana closed our time together with words of thanks and affirmation. Afterwards, several women came to speak to me, to hug me, to acknowledge what they had observed.

I believe my presence in the circle that day served a compelling purpose. For those last several minutes, I became a conduit to carry and contain the flow of emotional energy invoked by the ritual, a vivid display of our interconnectedness. The collective triggered what I see now as a luminous expression of grief over the loss of my mother and the long-delayed claiming of my menopausal self. I took with me an intense knowing that we move through these rites of passage both individually and together. We are not alone with our joys or our sorrows.

Endnotes

1. I described the origins of the concept of body literacy and its subsequent incursion into menstrual cycle and women's health discourse in the post "#bodyliteracy: a hashtag, a title, a meme?" which appeared on *Menstruation Matters*, the blog of Society for Menstrual Cycle Research.

Works Cited

Society for Menstrual Cycle Research. SMCR 2015 Program, p. 40, 28 May, 2015, issuu.com/jaxgonzalez/docs/smcr2015program. Accessed 9 Mar. 2021.

Wershler, Laura. "#bodyliteracy: a hashtag, a title, a meme?" *Menstruation Matters*, 28 July 2012, www.menstruationresearch.org/2012/06/28/bodyliteracy-a-hashtag-a-title-a-meme/. Accessed 7 Mar. 2021.

Wershler, Laura. "Charting My Way to Body Literacy." *Justisse, Winter 2006*, www.justisse.ca/MediaGallery/Femme%20Fertile/Femme%20Fertile%20Winter%202006.pdf. Accessed 7 Mar. 2021.

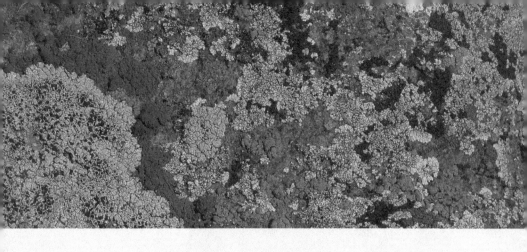

SECTION FOUR

UNLEASHED

Wherein women seize the freedom to be, to create, to push boundaries, and to disengage from expectations, societal norms, and assumptions about the aging reproductive body.

Chapter 14

Harsh Blessings:
On Finding Poetry at Fifty

Magali Roy-Féquière

Thirty-four and just married, we tried—to no avail—to get pregnant. With our Stanford doctorates in hand, and new jobs in the Midwest, my husband and I thought time was on our side. We were a hot couple, full of energy and ambition. After tenure, we would get down to the business of having a child. But no child came, so we headed for a fertility clinic in nearby Iowa City. I suspected that the blond, assisted-reproduction gynecologist had little interest in helping us conceive. Making conversation, he let on that he volunteered in Haiti, my country of birth. I was seven years old when we left the island. The Duvalier dictatorship had become intolerable, and in 1966, my parents made the wrenching decision to start again in neighbouring Puerto Rico. "Why go for high tech measures, when so many children need homes?" The question seeped from his gaze. I later found out that people like us have poor outcomes in fertility clinics. Was race a factor in our case? When I think back, doubt flutters. Was my attempt to gestate and mother a child some kind of excess?

Unassisted by technology, I got pregnant at forty-one and miscarried at eight weeks. I was vaguely prepared because the doctor could not find the heartbeat the week before. My body expelled the fetus in the faculty bathroom stall. It would take me fourteen years to tell my husband what I experienced that day. The details.

We were pioneers, those of us women getting doctoral degrees in the 1980s, I told a college friend recently. But this has been costly. She agreed. A brilliant lawyer, PhD, and editor of a big city Latino newspaper for years, she had come to motherhood in her late thirties and was raising a daughter. College-bound in the late 1970s, we could not have foreseen any of this. We had few models, but eagerly dove right into the pill, IUDs, legal abortions, higher education, and sexual freedom.

Menopause hit at fifty. It heightened my sense of body, renewing my sex drive. This was a disorienting, exciting, and sad time. I found myself eying younger men. Felt entrapped, bewildered. My husband took it in stride and did not ask embarrassing questions. But the uncertainty must have been discomfiting for him, too. My crisis was hormonal and expressed itself existentially and spiritually. I found meditation, started writing poetry, and became an intuitive photographer. I'm still a poet, but my photography remains amateurish, a means to an end, an attempt at eye training. Menopause dislodged something in my brain, a kind of rockslide inside my head. We are chemical beings, and, alas, the doors of perception are susceptible to buzzing pheromones taunting our senses. I started keeping deeply private journals, scribbling assiduously every day. There was a lot of crying.

A colleague my age studies sexual response in twenty-somethings. But there's an untapped motherlode of research possibilities elsewhere. What we need her to do is ask the army of middle-aged women on campus about our inner sexual and sensual lives. That last hormonal hurrah is a maelstrom of pleasure, pain, and fear. You realize that you miss your period. Your looks have changed, again. You struggle. Masturbation calms and frustrates. Those very close to you intuit that something is about to erupt. They keep silent vigil.

Off kilter during this time, I lost all interest in academic writing but still went to work everyday. Two women friends were my lifeline, as I wrote, wept, meditated, and spent a lot of energy at the gym. They were there for phone calls or coffee and held me in their hearts. Their kindness and tact helped me to keep it together. These women were the first readers of my poems. Astute and funny, they did not hold back their opinions of my work. One finally said, "I think you are getting better as a poet." We sometimes talked about how we treat time. As I struggled to accept my new body, they reminded me that I was not dead yet.

Before menopause, I had no idea I could create with words. The change forced me to slow down and realize that a different life was in front of me. I wrote in my journal: "If the poem is envisioned as an 'experiment of attention,' as Anne Waldman says,[1] it could help us voice subtle experiences without projecting the usual images that can dull our vision." The poems here are a result of the fresh perceptions that menopause thrust upon me. After bouts of weeping in the backyard, the shower, at my desk, I rediscovered ambition—an ambition that drives me to rewrite and reedit, to reimagine and expand, to get somewhere else with impressions and images, and to distill and extract something truthful. There is value in witnessing and discovering our changing tempos / elastic and mercurial / like the passing of summer / when you're seven / and time is everything and nothing.

Imago

She wakes up little by little
Doesn't know that she is bound
Silk threads

Sudden bursts of fever
at the throat, the head, the cunt
Thoughts turn liquid on her skin and eyes
Something is shifting

—Taste the fearsome, impossible beauty
of the chimera—

Poised at the edge of dread
Unsure her angles of vision and sensation
rainbows on her changed skin
Alien to ways once quotidian

Speech still beyond her tongue
her laughter explodes

—cougar, great mother, prune—

So little divulged about the purpose and truth
of shapeshifting

Still Life

Her heart brought low
by fears. She hated
the drooping her shoulders
assumed, imperceptible
relenting.
She had seen this before,
in women who dared not
step into the provinces
of their own choosing.

Cicatrice

The scalpel had sliced skin and muscles,
to make way for gloved hands, metal, lights.
There must have been discussions, lessons imparted,
visceral divinations.

She had been unconscious for their explorations.
But in the weeks that followed,
an animal aquatic and muscled overcame her
again and again as she slept.

Not having found what they went looking for,
they had packed her innards and closed
the pulsating and warm cavern,
satisfied that no malignancy was left behind.
Only a patched-up trail
from navel to pubic bone
that she retraced as she washed.

Endnotes

1. This idea, or point of view, is central to Anne Waldman's poetics. She has given a series a poetry workshops where she specifically develops this practice.

Works Cited

Waldman, Anne. "Dakini Poetics: Experiments of Attention." *Jewel Heart*, 14 Apr. 2012, www.jewelheart.org/wordpress/wp-content/uploads/2012/03/Dakini-Poetics_Experiments-of-Attention-A-Poetry-Workshop-with-Anne-Waldman-April-14-2012-JH-AA. pdf. Accessed 7 Mar. 2021.

Chapter 15

Uninhabitable Lives: Narrative Strategies of Menopause Experience in *Notes on a Scandal* and *Carol*

Sylvie Teillay-Gambaudo

Introduction

Leni Marshall proposes that "menopause serves to mark a turning point in women's aging" (x). Indeed, aging studies generally present menopause as what marks the change in a woman's life. Marshall's choice of the word "menopause" is typical of its use in aging studies, in medical narratives, and in popular accounts. Menopause is this umbrella term that refers to a wide variety of experiences pointing to different stages of a woman's life known as pre-, peri- and post-menopause. These terms do not refer to any definable moments, in the way a woman's first period definitely marks the onset of her fertile life. Perimenopause refers to a transitional life stage spanning several months or several years, a transition between nonmenopausal and menopaused. As such, perimenopause points to an area of experience with only approximate boundaries and unclear symptoms. As Ruth Formanek describes, menopause is marked by new processes, typically seen as symptoms, such as the fluctuation of follicle stimulating hormones (FSH), the failure to maintain a state of physiological stability, the failure to regulate temperature, moods or cognitive ability, and corporeal discomfort (80). But these events can also be symptoms of ills other than menopause (thyroid dysfunction, post-traumatic shock, or depression, for example) and cannot be said to define perimenopause strictly. So unlike other experiences women have in their lives (the onset of menses, for instance), menopause has the unique property of being a backwards-looking experience. As I have argued in "The Regulation of Gender in Menopause Theory," a woman can say for sure she was pre- or perimenopausal only once she has fulfilled the criteria for postmenopause, such as consistently high levels of FSH or one full year without menses (553). Definitions and theories of pre- and perimenopause are then formulated as retrospective accounts of what it felt like to be a woman during the years preceding menopause rather than here-and-now descriptions of experience. With perimenopause spanning anything up to ten years or more, women find themselves in a situation where more than a decade of personal experience is made of approximation and ambiguity. It is then a big part of a woman's life that is defined in such hazy terms. Studying the boundary that separates experience before menopause from life after (or more accurately with) menopause experience is, thus, particularly interesting if we seek to define the experience of what perimenopause feels like, or what philosophy would describe as a phenomenology of aging women.

If perimenopause is defined in hazy terms, we should, however, guard against agreeing to associate it with experiences of confusion and uncertainty, which is often the case in medical and popular practices. Indeed, the inability to successfully determine the boundary that separates experience before and after menopause—that is, the inability to define perimenopause as living experience—goes a long way to explaining how it comes to be associated with confused, uncertain states. Although it may happen that confusion is a marker of lived perimenopause, the experience of confusion and uncertainty is not only the symptom of perimenopause but also the outcome of medical and social epistemic[1] struggles at stabilizing the meaning of menopause. Hence, we should not accept that confusion and uncertainty are the trademark of perimenopause experience itself without argument. This is what I propose to do. In what follows, I will be using the term "menopause" to refer to both perimenopause and menopause experience without distinction. I hope it will become evident that drawing a distinction between perimenopause and menopause is a matter for medical semantics aimed at establishing menopause as a medical condition and perimenopause as a terrain of treatment rather than a narrative of what menopause actually feels like, which is what interests me here.

In this chapter, my aim is to unpack how we might represent the experience of women aging. In so doing, I am proposing from the start that the experience of aging cannot be dissociated from issues of gender. Strictly speaking, narratives of aging are not in themselves gender specific. Rather, they point to what is known as a "midlife crisis" in popular narratives. But if we compare women's narratives[2] with men's narratives of aging, it seems to me that men's narratives of aging are often more focused on the loss of sexual ability; such films as *American Beauty*, *Venus*, *Gran Torino*, *Sleeping Beauty*, or *Last Vegas* are all about virility and the battle against its loss to the aging process. Women's narratives of aging also incorporate sexuality. But I will argue that the loss of hegemonic understanding of sexual ability becomes an integral part of the way women navigate aging narratives successfully. Menopause narratives add a novel way of understanding aging by acknowledging loss as experience—a loss elicited by a changing body. In other words, menopause experience would be the opposite of a static experience arrested at what the body can no longer do, nor is it about how one might fight loss to recover one's former state of being. On the contrary, menopause experience would manifest itself as a continual transformative narrative of surrender to loss and the discovery of the new meanings it brings.

Menopause Narratives: Regulated and Obscured by Mainstream Narratives

What I am proposing to do is not new. There have been numerous attempts at establishing criteria that could constitute reliable definitions of menopause. In my earlier research on menopause ("Regulation of Gender"), I sought to situate menopause theories in relation to feminist interests. I found that, by and large, there are two broad frameworks— medical and evolutionary—that explain menopause experience. Regardless of their differences, these theories have in common epistemic premises founded on phallocentrism.

In theory, menopause should be that narrative that participates in a phenomenology of woman's experience and of woman only. In practice, phallogocentric[3] recuperation means that menopause has become an area of study that reenforces established narratives of gender. As I have argued: "Theories of menopause understand menopause experience in relation to the purpose woman serves in man's experience, for example: childcare, domesticity, disease. To challenge phallus-centred theories of menopause, one would need to theorize menopaused women's sensitive bodies, before or aside of mediation by men's perception of it (Gambaudo, "Regulation of Gender" 557).

To theorize "menopaused women's sensitive bodies" poses a problem, given that phenomenological narratives of menopause experience are dominated by narratives privileging the epistemic experience of males. Luce Irigaray has been highly successful at showing how the expression of human experience has been understood, in Western philosophy at least, as one dimensional. In 1985, she published her famous *Speculum of the Other Woman*, in which she describes what this one-dimensional vision of experience looks like. In her opinion, Western thought is incapable of accounting for the multiplicity of experiences. Dominant narratives of experience typically report experience that is mediated by the epistemic filter of men's rational thought. Irigaray believes that patriarchal phallocentric societies privilege men's experience to the point of being incapable of relating to experiences other than men's. That is, only those experiences mediated by men's own sensitive bodies and the rational understanding of those sensitive bodies can be intelligible. Hence, in a world mediated by men, women's experiences of uniquely female events, like pregnancy or menopause, become meaningful on the condition that they are framed against the gauge of men's sensitive understanding of those events—that is, the presence or absence of menstruation as evidence of the presence or absence of a man's impregnation. Furthermore, Irigaray contests logocentrism, which is the Western idea that there exists, as Schutte explains, a "transcendental subject of knowledge [who] coordinates and controls the multiplicity of sensations and impressions received from sense experience, thus forming a unified field of experience" (65). Logocentrism arrests the possibility of multiple truths, forcing the experience of ambiguity and uncertainty to become unified into a singular intelligible experience to be noticed and understood. Hence, narratives that would not seek to fuse scattered and conflicted elements of experience into a meaningful totality and that could typify aging experience cannot be heard.

In trying to understand what menopause is, then, dominant discourses (primarily medicine or evolutionary theory) have obscured what could have become more legitimate accounts of menopause (first-person accounts or scattered, conflicted narratives, for example) because menopause experience was mediated by male sensitivities, necessarily misguided in their apprehension of specifically female experience, and by men's interests, necessarily biased towards the advancement of men's cause. From the discovery of menopause,[4] the obscuring of legitimate accounts has been the terrain of scientific research, which was by and large a male realm until the 1970s.[5] Until then, definitions of menopause experience were what those male scientists perceived of women's experience of menopause—for example, that women are no longer fertile and that they experience physiological discomfort. Their conclusions were based on observation of women in comparison with aging men's experiences and in comparison with the same woman's younger incarnation of herself. In short, narratives of difference and loss typify definitions of menopause experience and inhibit other possible ones.

More concretely, medical and evolutionary accounts position menopause as that "area of experience that has become anomalous and no longer conforms to social recognition of woman" ("Regulation of Gender" 558). For example, infertility, mood swings, or vaginal dryness are all signs of faulty corporeal functions because they put collective interest in jeopardy; species survival, stability of self, or penetrative intercourse become, by contrast, the unspoken yet very real duties women can no longer fulfil once menopause has occurred. The challenge to phallogocentric telling of experience will then allow narrative to do two things: the reader/listener can recognize the dissenting narrative because it misfits the story of man's sensitive experience; the narrator/speaker actively dissents as soon as their terms of reference outside established epistemic frames of recognition.

Judith Butler suggests in *Bodies That Matter* that we could look at menopaused women's lives as "unlivable lives" or occupying social spaces that are "uninhabitable" (3). Unlivable lives are characterized by those experiences in which the individual becomes either injured or lost and cannot find a framework to grieve their experience because their lives were not recognized as viable, or lived, in the first place. In *Bodies*

That Matter, Butler typically focuses on the experience of AIDS, especially the experience of grief when someone loses a loved one to AIDS. Her findings are applicable to the menopause experience. Butler finds difficulty in grieving for the thousands who died because those lives were epistemically marked out by repression, even suppression. Given the normative social context driven by what Butler has coined as the "heteronormative matrix" in *Gender Trouble* (7), the dimorphising of gender into masculine and feminine, and of the sexed body into male and female, is the basis for producing individuals whose desires cannot be understood away from this epistemic matrix. In this context, gay men and menopaused women come to share a common ground of unintelligibility, as both groups are found lacking the ability to reinforce dimorphic markers: the ability to reproduce, the capacity to either impregnate or be impregnated. The outcome of lacking impregnability translates into feeling disenfranchised from conventional lifestyles. In reverse, disenfranchising oneself from conventional lifestyles becomes the means by which one may recapture a sense of epistemic agency. Resistance against epistemic bias suggests the ability to know what one is seeking disenfranchisement from. In the case of menopause, the possibility to grieve for one's premenopause life is possible on the condition that premenopaused women have a tangible object to mourn. This mournable object exists, provided a woman can recall from her past an image of herself that corresponds with hegemonic definitions of what constitutes a woman's livable life, for example as a wife or mother. The outcome of menopause is then either a recapturing of that livability, through medical solutions for example, or the grieving for one's past incarnation. In the second case, grieving one's once liveable life is concomitant with her moving to uninhabitable zones of experience and its expression.

While seeking cinematographic narratives of menopause experience, I was struck by how frequently aging experience was depicted alongside, or enmeshed with, other experiences that could be categorized as uninhabitable. In the next section, I discuss how the aging narratives in *Notes on a Scandal* and *Carol* are presented in a dynamic of mutual support with other narratives: criminality and aging on the one hand and homosexuality and aging on the other.

These other narratives (criminality and homosexuality) are epistemically loaded as uninhabitable zones of social experience and traditionally remain obscured by the demands of epistemic correctness. The direct consequence of the fall from grace that aging women experience allows them to share in an experience of disidentification with the status quo and to seek other epistemic practices of uninhabitable lives to bring their own menopause experience to light. In an unusual but logical partnering of marginal experience, aging narratives succeed in repopulating those deserted zones of being which were not that empty after all but merely not yet visible. What I would call "narrative partnering," thus, constitutes some form of method to render visible those uninhabitable experiences that menopause belongs to. I will also argue that the younger characters of *Notes on a Scandal* and *Carol* can and do choose to recapture their livability by occupying permitted spaces of experience while the older characters seek beyond grief to migrate and populate uninhabitable zones of social experience.

Repopulating Uninhabitable Experience: Associating Narratives with Other Outlaw Narratives

The two films chosen have in common a narrative depicting aging women in the process of grief for a past livability of experience, moderated by the discovery of new areas of experience once thought uninhabitable and the attempt to appropriate them.

Notes on a Scandal (hereafter *Notes*) tells the story of two women. Sheba Hart (Cate Blanchett) is a forty-something mother and wife. Born in a wealthy family and despised by her mother, she studies arts at university, where she meets her future husband, Richard (Bill Nighy), a lecturer considerably older than herself. She marries him young, has children, and becomes an arts teacher. We meet her when she joins a new school, where Barbara Covet (Judy Dench) teaches history. Barbara is a sixty-something single woman, living in a small flat with her cat. She is the narrator of the film, a sharp commentator who confines her often acerbic thoughts to a diary, making the title of the film. The intrigue is formed through the attraction each of them develops for someone younger than they—Sheba for her fifteen-year-old pupil, Steven (Andrew Simpson) and Barbara for Sheba. The scandal is about not only Sheba's pedophilic relationship with Steven but also Barbara's secret records of events and the way she gains control of Sheba's attention via blackmail.

Carol explores what we would today call a lesbian affair between

Therese (Rooney Mara), a young shop floor girl, and Carol (Cate Blanchett), a middle-aged wealthy woman in the process of divorce. The story is set in 1950s New York, a highly significant timeframe for film director Todd Haynes. As we will see, the period drama type of narrative, and 1950s America in particular, allow him to investigate the women's sexual desire in a context where it is at least reprehensible if not illegal. Hence, the narrative delves into the ways the narrator finds to disclose what must remain hidden, without falling into a crusade narrative about closeted desires and heroic comings-out.

Notes and *Carol* present some common characteristics in the manner aging is presented. Each narrative is initially driven by what appears as a discrepancy in the narrative of self—a discrepancy that can be directly tied to the aging experience. At the start of each story, the audience is made explicitly aware the aging characters have a definite ease at navigating their social environment. In *Notes*, the story begins with the headmaster collecting his staff members' reports on the functioning of each department and their suggestions for improvement. Barbara insolently undermines his action by producing a ridiculously short report of only a few lines while remaining comfortably serene before the silent stare of her appalled colleagues. Moreover, his objections are rebuffed with Barbara's arguments that expose his project as no more than a useless box-ticking exercise aimed at satisfying governmental bodies and policies rather than enhancing the pupils' learning experience. Barbara's comfortable defiance of authority figures comes with her age. She is close to retirement. She has not only done it all but also seen it all before, something that gives her the edge over younger colleagues, even if they are her hierarchical seniors. The headmaster's hopeful appeal for staff participation and his wish to do good are met with Barbara's assurance that what her short report says is "quite adequate" and more authentically reflects the social reality the school is facing.

Similarly, in the opening scenes of *Carol*, the main protagonist is a poised, mature woman, who is obviously wealthy and expects staff to facilitate her shopping experience. The audience gets a sense that her confidence also comes from her experience of life: She is married, her clothes denote her ostentatious wealth, and she is a master of social graces in the way she moves and speaks. But within a few minutes of displaying this self-assurance that comes with life gains, Carol also shows a more awkward facet of her character, when her expensive fur coat accidently

192

catches the lever that controls the toy train going in endless circles in front of Therese's workstation. Momentarily taken aback by her faux pas, she recomposes herself and leaves the scene. The camera lingers briefly on the empty space her departure causes. Hence, in this introductory scene, Carol is presented as the instrument of arrest of senseless and repetitive movement, leaving Therese (and the audience) with the spectacle of spatial emptiness instead.

In both films, the aging characters complain of feeling disenfranchised from life, and we witness their efforts at complying with social expectations of them: Barbara is slightly ridiculous in the excessive efforts she makes for Sheba's lunch invite. She splashes out on a new hairstyle, new clothes, and a big bouquet of flowers. On arriving at Sheba's, it becomes evident that her demeanour is totally at odds with Sheba's laid back, disorganized, and bourgeois bohemian lifestyle.

The loneliness and desolation of Barbara's life become palpable in her comments about the invite as "a merry flag on the Arctic wilderness of my calendar." As for Carol, part of the film's intrigue revolves around her separation and divorce. As she tries to negotiate the best terms possible for her and her child, self-imposed solitude and melancholy become key to placating her husband and his entourage. Hence, directors Richard Eyre (*Notes on a Scandal*) and Todd Haynes (*Carol*) offer us a discrepancy of self between what characters ought to be (i.e., facilitators of social occasions like family life) and what they actually are (i.e., characters with a secretive inner life that they do not feel entitled to live, let alone share with their entourage). The discrepancy becomes the opening through which Eyre and Haynes offer a critique of established narratives and new configurations of aging. Let us look at this critique a little closer.

In *Notes on a Scandal,* we are explicitly warned to "mind the gap." Sheba confides in Barbara her disappointment over what she has become: a facilitator of others' lives, such as the lives of her children, her husband, her pupils, and her friends. She appears resigned to her middle-aged condition. She describes her past life as a time when seduction and sexuality had centre stage—a life now exchanged for more sedate activities, like teaching and caring. But Barbara is from the start unconvinced about the victimized, awkward, and inadequate image that Sheba presents to the world: "Hard to read the wispy novice. Is she a sphinx or simply stupid?... A fey person I suspect.... Her voice is pure as if her mouth were empty and clean, as if she'd never had a filling." Barbara then clearly sees in Sheba the end of a narrative of self, a sphinx and fey, fated to die but also destined to resurrect from its ashes as something else. What Barbara cannot fathom is Sheba's desire. Does it match her own desire for the "spiritual recognition" shared with a companion that would have the ability "to see through the quotidian awfulness of things" or is Sheba a fake? Soon, Barbara uncovers that the latter is true. Sheba's desire is for a recapture of her former glory days, when husband Richard scooped her up and then left his wife and children for a nonstop "fuck fest." Barbara experiences Sheba's affair with pupil Steven as betrayal. Sheba's actions shatter Barbara's dreams for transformation and hope to inhabit those uninhabitable areas of experience discussed earlier. Sheba's betrayal is not that she has an affair but rather that she has an affair with a young man. Barbara feels betrayed on two fronts: one, because Sheba's choice of love object is a man and, second, because he is young. Sheba is rekindling her relationship with her "glory days," with the down and dirty business of "fuck fests," which signals her departure from Barbara's wish for "spiritual recognition." Spiritual recognition appears framed as lesbian desire, but I argue that if it is lesbian desire that animates Barbara, then it is a form of lesbianism that is not defined according to phallogocentric understandings of lesbianism.

The work of Julia Kristeva is useful here, as it proposes a different vision of lesbianism—one that is away from more consensual under-standings of homosexuality (as terrain of political activism for example). She partly proposes female homosexuality as aesthetic practice enabling the lesbian a way to challenge hegemonic forms of sexuality.[6] Kristeva's vision is, thus, particularly applicable to the context of this enquiry. Critiques (Toril Moi's for example) have traditionally associated the work of Kristeva with that of Irigaray (introduced earlier) for the way they position women's experiences in relation to phallus-centred epistemic frames. In the same way Irigaray has phallogocentrism at the centre of meaningful experience, Kristeva finds that to define (female) sexuality is always a question of situating it in relation to the symbolic framework. Sexual intelligibility is the domain of symbolic representation, and homosexuality is situated in the margin of that sexual intelligibility. Women's homosexuality is not in itself an epistemic narrative that is immediately available and meaningful. On the contrary, to find its specificity, we must turn to culturally coherent narratives formulated by approximation with already existing structures of sexual categories, for example, recognizing how butch/femme lesbian identities approximate masculine/feminine heterosexual ones. For Kristeva, true lesbianism is not the experiences of the woman-woman encounter but that of the feminine-feminine encounter, as she explains in *Interviews*. "In the end, recognizing feminine 'specificity' and 'creativity' associates them with the structures and identities borrowed from paternalistic and monotheistic societies. Because such societies do not recognize feminine specificity, they try to put it aside, subdue it, and make sure no one talks about it" (106). In the absence of a phallic signifier, the feminine-feminine encounter remains doubly unintelligible. In those terms, to define woman's homosexuality would be to find the modalities of the feminine-feminine encounter. In *Tales of Love* Kristeva, asks: "Could one imagine an erotics of the purely feminine?" (80). At first, the answer appears to be uncompromisingly "no": "To the extent that she has a loving soul, a woman is drawn into the same dialectic involving confrontation with the Phallus.... Whatever the organ, confrontation with power remains" (80-81).

If we return to *Notes*, Sheba closes the epistemic gap opened by her aging experience by having sex with Steven. The narrative implies an impossibility to find other ways for Sheba to navigate the gap created by the epistemic bias towards phallic representation, and she uses Steven's young, virile masculinity to signify the closure of her own sense of loss. What the film seems to imply is that to acknowledge herself as aging, a woman must either accept to fall out of the phallogocentric definition of sexual woman (she is now barren and/or desexualized) or reject such relegation and resist the parameters that place her there (hormone replacement therapy or plastic surgery, for example). Sheba chooses to reject relegation by having an affair with a male student. She, thus, temporarily rekindles her relationship with an image of herself that corresponds with phallogocentric sensibility.

Barbara, in contrast, chooses to embrace relegation to an uninhabitable experience. Possibly, the loss of sexual status translates into the loss of interest in phallus-centred sexuality. Barbara is searching for the right terms to define this other sexual narrative—a feminine-feminine type of lesbianism described by Kristeva in *Tales of Love* as "the delightful arena of a neutralized, filtered libido, devoid of the erotic cutting edge of masculine sexuality" (80-81). Barbara's desire to inhabit the uninhabitable could be framed as her desire for the feminine-feminine encounter, what she calls "spiritual recognition." She understands the potentiality of the bothersome gap as liveable space. For her secret diary, she reinvents herself as a condescending narrator, a savvy commentator of a world she obviously despises. A fearless character, she is a good teacher, an exemplary disciplinarian who cuts through the falsity of social situations with gusto, putting back in their places headmasters, colleagues, and pupils alike. But we get a sense of her that this is "the awfulness of things"—this is the masculine world she hopes to leave for spiritual recognition. To obtain spiritual recognition, Barbara believes she, and her coveted companion, need to see the gap and "the distance between life as you dream it and life as it is," a reckoning that emerges only with one's lived experience. In other words, only the acknowledgement of aging can bring the knowledge of the gap. As Sheba explains, the gap is the absence of meaning; it is the impossibility to bridge the divide between imagined and lived experience: an uninhabitable and uninhabited area of experience that Sheba is determined to not know and that Barbara serially attempts to inhabit.

The confrontation between the two models of aging (Sheba's and Barbara's) leads us to discouraging conclusions. Of the two, the one who seeks to hang on to a phallus-centred model of woman's experience appears to be the loser. Sheba's choice to stay with known experience is not presented as a happy ending. She is subjected to the violence of social organization, a violence that matches Sheba's own, as she is losing what she was. When she emerges into the crowd of journalists, looking dishevelled, her face intentionally smeared with dark make-up, screaming a defiant "Here I am!" it is not just the monstrosity of her pedophile act that she throws at the excited crowd of journalists but also the monstrosity of what she is becoming by virtue of aging: somebody whose story is beginning to derail and is increasingly defined as what she no longer is. Sheba quickly disappears from the narrative after this, and we only get a mention of her starting a prison sentence towards the end of the film.

Barbara seems to fare better. However, as Sheba's unravelling unfolds, we discover that Barbara's attempt at finding spiritual recognition is not that different from Sheba's strategy. Barbara has done this before, and by the end we know she will do it again. Her predation on women younger than herself is uncomfortably reminiscent of Sheba's avoidance strategy. As Barbara gets satisfaction from the predation of younger women, her desire to inhabit aging experiences, off the radar of phallogocentric representations of desire, is doomed to fail because she herself endorses a phallogocentric position with the different women she encounters. By the end of *Notes*, we are in no doubt as to the outcome of her predation of Annabelle (Anne-Marie Duff), Barbara's new contender for spiritual recognition.

Could then finding the terms to narrate a nonphallic sexual experience become the challenge of menopause narratives? Given the hierarchy of meaning of phallus-centred expression, we find that narratives aiming to dissociate from this hierarchy are positioned on the side of the marginal, even as nonintelligible creation. It is then no surprise that we should find narratives of menopause associated with other marginal or nonsensical narratives, for example that of homosexual desire. The motives are multiple. For one, it is to do with the difficulty in finding a comprehensible framework to relate the experience of aging. The medicalization of menopause experience remains the closest available discourse for its formulation. But save for wanting to frame a story of aging women in medical terms, the next available pathological framework (i.e., homosexuality) helps the narrator superimpose pathology and dissent in a manner that makes the illegitimacy of aging narratives immediately plain. *Notes* tells us of the possibility of such narratives, which in the film appear to fail. The narrative of *Carol* alludes to similar difficulties but with more successful outcomes for the aging woman of the film.

The setting of *Carol* in early 1950s America becomes part of the story's intrigue and provides the director with a strategy to make obvious the collusion of different narratives. The 1950s have a particular place in Haynes's work (see *Far From Heaven,* also set in the 1950s), as loyalty to the period drama motif obliges the narrator to respect the rigid behavioural codes of the time. In the 1950s, New York was a place where homosexuals were persecuted through what was known as the "lavender scare," a government-led witch hunt designed to cleanse government civil service of homosexuality. Homosexuals were portrayed as individuals posing security risks, often accused of communist sympathies, which shows how much the lavender scare was imbued with the McCarthyistic anticommunist spirit that animated the United States between 1950 and 1956 (Johnson). The representation of unlivable experience is then an exercise in finding expression that befits the 1950s motif: subtly disguised rather than loudly declared. Haynes closely adheres to Phyllis Nagy's 1997 adaptation of Patricia Highsmith's 1952 novel.[7] In the film, we find that Carol's intelligibility as a divorcee, mother, and homosexual is dependent upon establishing her life experience as pathology. The character embarks on a course of psychotherapy, which, we later learn from her therapist's report, is aimed at reinserting Carol on the legally and socially acceptable side of divorce and motherhood—that is, as a celibate, sacrificial, and unfulfilled character, key characteristics of a 1950s phallocentric perception of women, divorcees, and homosexuals.

Carol clearly plays with the contrast between visible compliance to social codes and discreet transgression of conformity in moments that appear suspended, as if springing from a parallel world that the women also inhabit. Haynes used different means to make that transgressive journey evident. The relationship between the two women is played out in a way that made some critics describe it as "cold," even "chilly" (Sims), for the lack of demonstrative intimacy on the one hand and, on the other, the concealment of intimacy within the fabric of the permitted text. The permitted text is located in the mundane exchanges, civilities, and polite conversation, while intimacy remains hidden from view, only just perceptible behind the 1950s decorum. In what could be termed intimacy of the shallow, Haynes (and with him, cinematographer Edward Lachman) succeeds in capturing a concealed narrative—one that runs alongside the 1950s text and that is perceptible in the audio-visual layer of the story. The scene where Carol picks up Therese in her car to take her on a visit to her country house is a strong example. There is a superimposition of several layers of representation, enmeshed with and disrupting the 1950s type of narrative. The mundane (shallow, even clichéd vignettes of the 1950s) is muffled, whereas the specifics (intimate details extracted from those vignettes) are magnified. We cannot hear conversations, presented as background noise, as the scene is covered by an eerie music that delays its notes and conveys a sense of anticipation, withholding, and apprehension. The musical score becomes one of the overlaid narratives that contributes to the expression of the transgressive text. The composer of the film score, Carter Burwell, describes how he drowned the auditory space with an abundance of notes heard as if distorted by spatial resonance (*Carol*, DVD Special Features). Haynes, thus, clearly aims to confuse narrative expectations by manipulating auditory and visual fields. To return to the scene in the car, the camera comes out of focus when filming a general view of the scene and goes into focus when pointing at odd details. The effect is of a blurred scenery, the contours of which cannot be discerned, compelling the audience to concentrate on the sharper details. The entire screen is occupied with the moving of Carol's lips while she is speaking an inaudible speech or with the shape of her jaw or with the movement of her gloved fingers on the radio controls as it plays a 1950s love song heard as if from a distance. These are all magnified elements, pulled out of the broad picture—details that Therese is bringing into focus in an internalized, secret narrative of what it is like to fall in love and that the audience is invited to share. In other scenes, like the final scene between Carol and Therese, Haynes achieves a similar effect not only by bringing the world out of focus but also by slowing down its motion, all the while focusing on the immobility of his characters and the restrained minute changes in their facial expression. Finally, throughout the film, the colour red is reserved for one or two objects per scene (Therese's woolly hat or Carol's nail varnish for example), contrasting with the overall restrained grey and beige colours that dominate the replica 1950s colour pallet.

Hence, the manipulation of different dimensions of narrative—including the audio, visuals, and timeframe—allows for a reversed focus effect, whereby the general dominant view becomes background scenery for the unfolding of subdued, discreet moments of intimacy between the two protagonists, the persistence of which gives the impression of a continuous narrative that cuts through phallogocentric representation of the 1950s experience. In a twenty-first-century world, where individuals are encouraged to publicly declare their feelings to each other and on social media, the perceived coldness of the characters has more to do with the difficulty that some viewers face in imagining a world where experience cannot be spelled out and remains outlawed— visible only through the fabric of the broader narrative.

Conclusions

If a definition of older women's desires cannot be established because those desires are obscured by the regulatory forces required by patriarchal narratives of menopause experience—from perimenopause to postmenopause—it does not mean its telling is impossible. On the contrary, the narratives of *Notes on a Scandal* and *Carol* present narratives where the (re)sexualization of older women takes centre stage. They have in common a narrative strategy that encodes the telling of the aging woman's story within the context of other recognized narratives of marginal experience. The one I have chosen to highlight is homosexual desire, but I have also alluded to more discrete ones, such as narratives of criminality, mundane environments, and volatile systems of meaning. My point is that narratives of older women's desires navigate the same strategies of meaning as other narratives that typically struggle to find social acceptance, such as extramarital love or homosexual love. I have described how *Notes on a Scandal* and *Carol* use marginal narratives of homosexual desire to cash in on their success at explaining what marginality feels like, away from established conclusions of doom and gloom. *Notes* fails to fully account for Barbara's (and Sheba's) aging experiences; nevertheless, it proposes an interesting contrast between two attempts at navigating the experience of aging and what aging feels like to the protagonists.

Whereas *Notes* stops at phallogocentric short-sightedness, *Carol* goes further and offers the viewer a narrative of aging in which the protagonists come out of obstruction and find epistemic strategies to go beyond it. As in *Notes*, the collision between the two choices is also clearly spelled out in *Carol*; the moment Carol leaves Therese is the moment the protagonists attempt to shift epistemic tactics. We see how Carol's pathologizing of her situation is the means by which she hopes to regain access to her position as a mother. In a dramatic scene, she decides to forego custody of her child: "I have no clue what is best for me. But I do know, and I feel it in my bones what is best for my daughter.... What use am I to her ... if I am going against my own grain?" Carol foresees a bleak future for herself and her daughter, who will be mothered by someone whose life has been pushed to the margin of acceptability and whose existence will remain conditional upon good behaviour (demonstrating celibacy, sacrifice, and lack of fulfilment). She, thus, opts to embrace that margin. Is this to say *Carol* offers a successful narrative of aging? Not if by successful we mean some authentic narrative of self that was always already there for the protagonists to discover and that they triumphantly find and proclaim. On the contrary, *Carol*'s narrative of aging is contained in those few words that Carol writes to Therese: "Please don't be angry when I tell you [that] you seek resolutions and explanations because you're young, but you will understand this one day. And when it happens…. I want you to imagine me there to greet you." Aging, then, is about giving up on finding resolutions and explanations for the changeability of life. Embracing uncertainty as well as inhabiting uninhabitable spaces would be its overarching theme. Therese initially comes out of her heartbreak more adult, more mature, and more apt at making the choices that will keep her on the correct side of being. But again, Haynes shows Therese's choice as background noise to a silenced story. Therese is seen resisting the terms of this silent narrative over and over again: when she receives a note from Carol inviting her to a meeting and categorically crumples the note and bins it or when she meets Carol again and refuses to rekindle the relationship or when she goes to a party and struggles to fit in. In each of these scenes, we also see her failing to reach closure, failing to gain certainty: She throws the note away but goes to the meeting; she rejects Carol's advances but is visibly shaken by Carol's departure, mimicking the opening scenes of their first encounter, where Carol left an empty space where she once stood; and at the party, she visibly does not fit in and leaves early. The film closes with a scene in which we are led to believe that she returns to Carol, choosing to inhabit unlivable spaces again.

So, how shall we conclude? The two films I have presented were chosen because they offer a similar narrative of aging with differing conclusions. Both depict aging women confronted with the loss of social significance at the point when their sexual abilities are put into question. I suggested at the start that a true narrative of women aging would not seek to fuse scattered and conflicted elements of experience into a meaningful totality. At the end of my study, I find that *Carol* is more successful than *Notes* at achieving this. Although *Notes* suggests Barbara's ongoing resistance, in the relationship between her and Annabelle, the narrative is also framed in the context of Barbara's moral wrongdoing: She prompted Sheba's downfall and at the end feels no remorse, no compassion, and certainly no love for Sheba. In fact, Sheba's demise, now a newspaper front-page topic, becomes instrumental in Barbara's seduction of Annabelle, when Barbara brags about the fact that she personally knew Sheba, exciting the interest of her young and naïve new friend. We know how their story will go. Hence, in *Notes*, there is a sense of totalization in the form of Barbara's deviousness. The narrative is totalized in the manner it points to and distances itself from outlaw narratives—those that phallogocentrism does not allow or recognize as valid. The personal narrative of aging is, thus, spelled out and is supported by the clear positioning of the bad (i.e., immorality) on the side of the aging women (Sheba for pedophilia and Barbara for inflicting psychological harm). In other words, *Notes* gives us a glimpse of phallogocentric short-sightedness, only to recoil from it and warn us against it.

Carol goes further. It offers the viewer a narrative of aging in which the protagonists come out of obstruction, and the narrative successfully presents epistemic strategies to go beyond obstruction. The key is in who makes choices in the end. Carol, the aging woman, comes to resist the terms of a divorce that would condemn her to conceal her experience. She invites Therese to join her but is rebuffed by the younger woman. Therese is young, she is socially attractive, and she is on the way to a successful career: It is clearly her moment. Because her life ticks the boxes of social success, her choice to resist hegemonic narrative is all the more noticeable; she has no valid reason to choose otherwise. The film ends on the subtle smile of Carol when Therese approaches. Because the story of Carol and Therese has already been told, the audience does not need to imagine the terms of the relationship. Here again, they already know. But there is no sense of closure, no totalizing effect in Haynes's narrative strategy because there is no triumph over adversity. Therese is embracing uncertainty, choosing to inhabit uninhabitable spaces. So, there is no heroic triumph, but there is Todd Haynes's aesthetic accomplishment, showing us beyond valid reason how narratives of resistance may be done and enjoyed. At the end of *Carol*, the terms by which one obstructs hegemonic experience are no longer exclusive to a particular experience. It is not just about aging or just about homosexuality or just about 1950s America. But it is about the reversal of expected narratives, when epistemic correctness, which requires one to keep certain experiences obscured, becomes the background noise to new narratives of personal experience. In this sense, Haynes's achievement could be recuperated for more than aesthetic ends. It also hints at political impact by highlighting the transformative power of women's experience to navigate and find strategies of meaning that render visible those experiences that social conventions conceal.

Endnotes

1. I will use the term "epistemic" as a shortcut to refer to the manner in which a word gains validation founded on a predefined understanding and knowledge of what experience the word points to. In this study, the use of the word "menopause," and associated ones like "perimenopause," points to the difficulty in defining a phenomenology of aging women's experience because the epistemic understanding of aging women is mediated by the experience and knowledge of men and/or that of medical science, whether the experience is voiced by a man or a woman.

2. I will use *Notes on a Scandal* and *Carol* here, but other films share similar narrative patterns, *The Page Turner* or *The Gymnast* for example.

3. The term phallogocentrism, coined by Irigaray, is a contraction of three terms: phallus, logos, and centrism. Phallogocentrism describes the epistemic difficulty of accounting for women's experience. Western thought is invested in the creation and maintenance of narratives that only report on the experience of man and on its incapacity to account for other experiences. When we apply this idea to menopause experience in phallocentric (phallus-centred) societies, like Western societies, we find that menopause experience becomes intelligible only on the condition that it echoes man's sensitive experience of menopause (e.g., medical discourse), and that the terms by which this experience is described have already become established and are, thus, recognized as menopause experience.

4. The existence of menopause is recorded as far back as biblical times (e.g., Abraham and Sara). But we have to wait until the eighteenth century for a more objective, scientific definition of menopause to emerge (Formanek 448).

5. Although there were many pioneer female doctors, it is only from the 1970s that we see a true change in the male-female doctor ratio in the Western world. I do not have the space to elaborate on this fascinating area of gender medicine, but we can attribute this shift in attitudes to a combination of factors, notably changes in the political climate ("Women in Medicine") and the impact of the political work of second-wave feminists (Paludi et al.).

6. Kristeva's vision of lesbianism includes the lesbianism of males, especially of male artists. (see my "Julia Kristeva, 'Woman's Primary Homosexuality,' and Homophobia").

7. Patricia Highsmith's novel, *The Price of Salt*, was published by Coward-McCann in 1952 under the pseudonym Claire Morgan. It was reprinted in 1990 under the title *Carol* by Bloomsbury. Phyllis Nagy adapted the novel for film in 1997. This script, directed by Todd Haynes, was finally brought to the screen in 2015.

Works Cited

Butler, Judith. *Bodies That Matter: On the Discursive Limits of "Sex."* Routledge, 1993.

Butler, Judith. *Gender Trouble*. Routledge, 2008.

Carol. Directed by Todd Haynes, Studio Canal, 2015.

Formanek, Ruth. *The Meanings of Menopause: Historical, Medical and Clinical Perspectives*. New York and London: Routledge, 1990.

Far From Heaven. Directed by Todd Haynes, Universal Pictures Home Entertainment, 2003.

Gambaudo, Sylvie. "The Regulation of Gender in Menopause Theory." *Topoi: An International Review of Philosophy*, vol. 36, no. 3, 2017, pp. 549-59.

Gambaudo, Sylvie. "Julia Kristeva, 'Woman's Primary Homosexuality,' and Homophobia." *European Journal of Women's Studies*, vol. 20, no. 1, 2011, pp. 8-20.

Gran Torino. Directed by Clint Eastwood, Warner Bros, 2008.

Highsmith, Patricia. *The Price of Salt*. Dover Publications, 2015. Originally published in 1952 under the pseudonym Claire Morgan by Coward-McCann. Reprinted in 1990 under the title *Carol* by Bloomsbury.

Irigaray, Luce. *Speculum of the Other Woman*. Cornell University Press, 1985.

Johnson, David, *The Lavender Scare: The Cold War Persecution of Gays and Lesbians in the Federal Government*. University of Chicago Press, 2006.

Kristeva, Julia. *Julia Kristeva Interviews*, edited by Ross Mitchell Guberman, and translated by Suzanne Clark and Kathleen Hulley, Columbia University Press, 1996.

Kristeva, Julia. *Tales of Love*. Columbia University Press, 1987.

Last Vegas, Directed by Jon Turteltaub, CBS, 2013.

Marshall, Leni. "Aging: A Feminist Issue." *Women's Studies Association Journal*, vol. 18, no. 1, 2006, pp. vii-xiii.

Notes on a Scandal. Directed by Richard Eyre, Fox Searchlight Pictures, 2006.

Schutte, Ofelia. "Irigaray and the Problem of Subjectivity." *Hypatia*, vol. 6, no. 2, 1991, pp. 64-76.

Paludi, Michele, et al. *Foundations for a Feminist Restructuring of the Academic Disciplines.*, 1990.

Sims, David. "Why *Carol* Is Misunderstood." *The Atlantic*, 15 Jan. 2016, www.theatlantic.com/entertainment/archive/2016/01/carols-misunderstood-coldness/424419/. Accessed 21 Feb. 2017.

Sleeping Beauty. Directed by Julia Leigh, Paramount Pictures, 2011.

The Gymnast. Directed by Ned Farr, Warner Bros, 2006.

The Page Turner (La Tourneuse de page). Directed by Denis Dercourt, Artificial Eye, 2006.

Venus. Directed by Roger Michell, Miramax, 2006.

"Women in Medicine: A Review of Changing Physician Demographics." *Staff Care*, 2015, www.staffcare.com/women-in-medicine-changing-physician-demographics-white-paper/?mobile=0. Accessed 13 Sept. 2017.

Chapter 16

Perimenopause: The Body, Mind, and Spirit in Transition

Victoria Team

In the middle of my journey through perimenopause, my perception of it has changed profoundly. I used to think it was just a nuisance—a time when women have hot flushes, night sweats, irritability, and irregular periods before they stop menstruating. I thought that it was a life-stage transition that all women would easily go through, although less patient women might rely on hormone replacement therapy. Perimenopause has been defined as "the period of time before and for a year after the final menstrual period during which time ovarian hormonal patterns, experiences and sociocultural roles change" (Zala, Swan, and Prior 252). Additionally, for the purposes of this chapter, I define it as the period of noticeable or non-noticeable changes in my body, mind, and spirit related to these complex hormonal and sociocultural changes.

I describe myself as a white, middle-class woman who is in a mixed marriage with a man of African background. I am a mother of five and a grandmother of four. I trained as a medical doctor in Ukraine, which at the time was part of the former Soviet Union, and I lived and practiced in Africa for ten years. I then immigrated with my family to Australia, where I completed my postgraduate degrees in public health. Therefore, I discuss the perimenopausal transition as a woman, a health professional, and a researcher. Autoethnography, as a method, allows me to bring these perspectives together. Andrea O'Reilly has noted that "first-person accounts" may improve our understanding of women's roles and their health issues (xv), and Sue Ziebland and colleagues have written that interest in other people's personal experiences is increasing, given that "traditional health information has been based on facts and figures and not on patient experience" (v). Expanded knowledge, improved understanding of patients' perspective, and appropriate translation strategies are the basic foundations for change and the main facilitators for quality improvements in healthcare (Coulter 13).

In the research on menopause, women's experiences of menopausal transition are frequently dichotomized. Biomedical researchers have focused on the negative aspects they research and write about, focusing mostly on hormonal changes as well as related symptoms and syndromes (Gordon, Beatty, and Whelan-Berry 919). Feminist researchers, meanwhile, have focused on social changes and argue that some women have positive or at least neutral experiences (Dillaway, "Menopause Is the 'Good Old'" 399). The menopausal transition has been described as a bio-psycho-socio-cultural transition (Hunter and Rendall 261). However, less attention has been paid to the spiritual component among the multiple psycho-socio-cultural factors. The need for a holistic model of the menopause transition, in addition to the biomedical and social models, has emerged. Margaret Harris defines the holistic model as reflecting "connections and interconnections, where the whole person is implicated through biological, psychological, emotional, and spiritual connections" (968), which can only be evident in women's personal accounts of the menopausal transition. Women's experiences are different; women may have positive and negative experiences at the same time, which have also been described as idioms of distress and normality (Salis et al. 520). The timing of the onset and the end of this transition is also different (Gold 425).

There is no consensus regarding the stages of the menopausal transition, which causes confusion and frustration for women, health professionals, and researchers. Referring to this transition, Heather Dillaway writes that "It is still difficult to know what experiences actually fall within this process, when it starts and ends, and how long it lasts" ("When Does Menopause Occur" 40). Whereas some people clearly identify only three stages—including perimenopause, menopause, and post menopause—others include some substages, such as early and late perimenopause, and argue that this transition has five or seven stages

(34). In my autoethnographic experience of the perimenopausal period, I clearly identify these substages. Discussing early, mid, and later stages of perimenopause, I focus on changes in my social circumstances followed by changes in my body, mind, and spirit. I also highlight various approaches that I applied to manage these changes.

Early Perimenopause

In my early forties, I entered into the early stage of perimenopause, which lasted about seven years. My periods decreased from seven to five days and became less heavy. Through this early phase, I did not experience the common negative perimenopausal symptoms, such as hot flushes, sweats, and disrupted sleep patterns. I did notice some changes in my behaviour, which I now, looking back, attribute to the early perimenopause (Zala, Swan, and Prior 26). This stage was one of the happiest in my life, coinciding with positive changes in my family and social circumstances. I finished my doctoral degree. I was on sessional contract teaching a few tutorial groups of medical students. I had more time for gardening and housework. We purchased a new house in a quiet, prestigious suburb. My oldest daughter had married and lived separately. My other two were enrolled in university courses. My older son had started secondary school and the youngest was in primary. They did not require as much care as when they were younger.

I enjoyed life and the activities I was involved with. I did everything with passion. I gardened and washed clothes in the morning. In the afternoon, after folding dried clothes, I cooked. On Wednesdays, when my husband was at work, my older kids came home on their own. I picked up my youngest son from school myself, on foot, because he loved to walk home rather than drive. We both enjoyed the extra time together, and he looked forward to playing on the swings and slides of the playground we passed through on our way home. Being able to mother more fully after submitting my thesis led to happiness. My parents lived with us. Although my father had had multiple hip and knee surgeries, he was able to do most activities either independently or with minimal support. My mother helped me manage household activities. We were a typical "sandwich" family.

I felt happy and excited. I became a bit childish, as one of the Dillaway's participants also explained ("Menopause Is the 'Good Old"

409), comparing her perimenopausal experiences with her teenage experiences. I enjoyed listening to music, dancing, and exercising. I purchased a skipping rope, as I had enjoyed skipping as a child. Other changes in my identity were reflected in my hobbies and interests. My passion for collecting Russian dolls and Ukrainian Easter eggs faded, and I started collecting Greek urns and plates instead, followed by Jewish menorahs and Israeli brass vases. My husband occasionally brought home vases from antique shops—thoughtful gifts that proved he was paying attention.

For a while, I attended Greek cultural events and festivals; later, I attended Messianic Jewish celebrations. I was aware that menopausal transition is culturally shaped and that the "notion of a universal menopause" was challenged (Lock and Kaufert 494). However, I did not come across studies discussing shifts from one cultural identity to another occurring during this transition, although I realize these shifts are most likely to occur in women from mixed ethnic and cultural backgrounds.

I found time for pot painting, something I had always wanted to do. I purchased terracotta pots and urns from local markets and secondhand shops. I used oil paint mixed with linseed oil to paint either black-and-red images, similar to images on Ancient Greek vases and plates, or colourful African images. The images ranged from erotic to religious, reflecting my perimenopausal state. Some were related to my mixed identity and to women's life in general. A few photographic images of these pots were published in books and journals. As discussed in the literature, through menopausal transition, women have often changed their hobbies or had more time for their hobbies (Gordon, Beatty, and Whelan-Berry 335).

I became more concerned about how I looked. I changed clothing styles, purchased jewelry, and tried various haircuts and hair colours. I wanted to be attractive. I appreciated and sought compliments. This desire was so strong that I actively tried to attract people to whom I was not attracted myself and with whom I did not want any kind of relationship. From an introvert, bookworm, and nerd, and also a religious person who adhered to the rules of Christian modesty—a housewife who, for most of my life, did not change my stay-at-home-mum outfit for days at a time—I turned into a shamelessly seductive Cleopatra. I did not simply walk past people, I showed myself, as if to say: "Look at me and send me your compliments." Rahele Samouei and Mahboubeh Valiani found that during this life stage, some Iranian women wanted to invite guests to their homes on a more frequent basis, aiming "to attract their attention" and "to show" themselves to their guests (e2).

As a Christian, I was concerned with my behaviour to attract people, particularly of the opposite sex. I recalled my grandma's instructions to me when I was a teenager: "If you attract boys, they will lust for you, and lust is a sin." She read me Matthew 18:7: "Woe to the world because of the things that cause people to stumble! Such things must come, but woe to the person through whom they come!" I asked God's forgiveness for my changed behaviour, but I still did everything to be attractive.

I did not consider these behaviours to be perimenopausal signs. Yet I noticed that my kids started using the words "menopausal" and "perimenopausal" when they were describing my style or activities. For example, "Mum, why have you planted flowers of all possible colours? Your garden looks perimenopausal." They made me realize that some of my activities did not correspond well with my age and that there was something odd about me doing things like skipping. My clothing style changed, but I perceived myself neither as a lady "growing old gracefully" (264) nor as "mutton dressed as lamb" (262)—the common social constructs of perimenopausal women described by Eileen Fairhurst. My approach was dress to impress. My daughters critiqued all my outfits, including casual outfits worn at home. When I wore leggings and jeans mini-skirt, they told me I looked like a "twelve-year-old bogany slut." In Australia, "bogan" usually refers to an unfashionable person of low socioeconomic status. When I wore a red t-shirt with starfishes and other marine creatures, they said I looked like a "waitress from the French seafood restaurant they visited while on holidays." When I put on a black pencil skirt and orange top, they told me I looked like a "JetStar flight attendant." They bought clothes they believed would suit me. My oldest daughter regularly supplied me with shoes and French cosmetics. My middle daughter purchased a navy pencil dress and red shoes and said, "This outfit is age appropriate, but you would still look sexy." My youngest daughter on one occasion bought me five pairs of slim-fit jeans in different colours. I appreciated their generosity and their funny comments and suggestions regarding my style.

Midstage Perimenopause

The excitement and happiness of early-stage perimenopause did not last. In my late forties, my family circumstances changed. Over a six-month period, I had a miscarriage, my mum had planned surgery, my husband had four surgeries requiring general anesthesia, and my father, in advancing ill health, died. I stayed with each family member in different hospitals, and if allowed to stay overnight, I slept on a chair or marked student assignments. Pregnancy loss, extensive caregiving, parental loss, and related grief contributed to my physical exhaustion, emotional distress, fatigue, and lack of enthusiasm. I described these health states as midlife burnout—a concept I've defined elsewhere "as a combination of mothering, marital, caregiving, perimenopausal, reproductive, and professional burnouts" (Team 148).

I became pregnant at forty-eight. When my period was eight weeks late, my husband and I first thought that it was the beginning of the perimenopausal transition. Although we did not plan to conceive, we were both happy to see the two lines in the results window of the pregnancy test. We were happy to have another child because we considered children a gift from God, although we had a clear expectation of our reduced chances to have a baby at my age. I had no major health issues, and I was feeling well but, unfortunately, I miscarried. I attributed the postmiscarriage changes in my body, mind, and spirit—such as tachycardia, mild uterine cramps, painful breasts, sore nipples, breastmilk production, accompanied with hot flashes and sweats, weakness, anxiety, depression, sadness, tearfulness, and hopelessness— to miscarriage rather than to perimenopause. However, most of these changes and signs, including the miscarriage, are related to perimenopause.

My husband comforted me, saying that we might have another child, but I became concerned that I may have lost my reproductive capacity. Something powerful compelled me to try to get pregnant again. As early as two months postmiscarriage, I attempted to calculate my ovulation days in order to conceive again to prove my ability to have a child. Our sexual interaction changed from enjoyable to purely biological, just to conceive. After a couple of months of unsuccessful attempts, I started to use these calculations as a contraceptive method out of fear of my age-related increased risk of chromosomal abnormalities and pregnancy complications. But then again, after a couple of cycles of contraception, we tried to conceive, asking God to bless us with a healthy child. These alternating conception-contraception cycles contributed to my exhaustion. My husband's surgeries, increased caregiving commitments, and the death of my father brought me to my senses: I abandoned my intention to conceive.

During this time, my periods became heavier and more frequent. Heavy bleeding is relatively common in perimenopause and is referred to as "flooding" episodes, when women experience a strong and continuing flow (Prior 538). "Tsunami" best describes the flow of my own changed periods, as it came in waves several times a day. Maternity-size pads, even supported with my husband's old t-shirts wadded up between my legs, did not have the capacity to hold the volume. Once at a social gathering in a café, I had a hot flush and dizzy spell, felt a massive uterine wave, and noticed a stream of blood running through the mesh chair to the floor. Embarrassment exacerbated my perimenopausal signs. I was red faced and sweaty; my heart was pounding. One thought consumed me: How do I cover up my perimenopausal mess? I first stepped in the small puddle of blood to hide it and then wiped it up with soft tissues I found in my bag. I covered the large red spot on the chair with the only thing at hand: my snow-sparkling cloth napkin. Fortunately, I was wearing a black skirt, so I hoped the blood stain was not noticeable. To reassure myself, I placed the strap of my bag over my shoulder and moved the bag around to my back to cover the spot. I discussed with my daughters my intention to offer payment to the café manager for the chair and the napkin. They discouraged me from doing this, with one saying: "Mum, they are well covered for all possible damage. Also, how will you provide your explanation if the café manager is a man?"

I first experienced the tsunami wave the morning after my father's death. It started with a severe and painful episode of diarrhea that left me feeling as if the epithelial lining had been ripped from my guts. It was accompanied by a flush, dizziness, and heart palpitations. For a few moments all I saw was black. I somehow managed to turn on the cold water, wash my face, and have a sip of water. When I was able to see again, I found myself standing in a puddle of blood. I thought that I had caught a gastro-intestinal infection from the hospital ward where I was looking after my father and that this viral infection also had affected my period. Ever since, I have had severe and repeated episodes of diarrhea prior to and in the early days of my periods. It took me some time to notice this link and to realize this was my body's reaction to changing estrogen, progesterone, and cortisol levels.

I started to have severe palpitations experienced as irregular heartbeats and a fluttering in my chest that lasted up to several minutes. Three times I was taken by ambulance to the emergency department, followed by admission to hospital and referral to a general practitioner (GP). The doctors were unable to determine the cause. They related this symptom to a chest infection. I remember my cardiologist saying that although he was not sure about the cause of the palpitations, he was certain there was nothing wrong with my heart. He suggested I do a cardiac stress test to exclude ischemic heart disease. At the time of these hospital emergency visits and hospital admissions, I had five chest x-rays to rule out chest infection and four electrocardiograms (ECGs) to rule out a cardiovascular event. My x-rays were clear, but as one of the doctors explained, "They may not show changes in the beginning of infection." Instead of a diagnosis, I had an ECG finding: sinus tachycardia. On one occasion, the emergency room doctor recommended an MRI. His suspicion that I had a pulmonary blockage was not confirmed by this test.

Frequently, I would wake up because my heart was fluttering. One of the GPs I saw prescribed Temazepam, a drug used to treat short-term sleeping problems, even though I told him I had no trouble sleeping. I was worried that I might develop a benzodiazepine dependence, and for a few nights, I took half of the prescribed dose. It knocked me out, but my palpitations did not disappear. I reduced the dose to one quarter of the tablet, which I took for another few nights before deciding not to take these tablets any longer.

During the palpitations, my blood pressure would usually increase, either because of hormonal changes or the accompanying anxiety. My blood pressure monitor and Littmann stethoscope were always at hand. Although I did not keep a diary of my blood pressure records, I noticed that on some days and weeks, I had normal blood pressure. On the day when my palpitations were particularly frequent and prolonged and my heart rate and blood pressure increased, I went to see another GP. I told him I was taking Temazepam and it was not helping. I also told him I did not take the whole dose because I was worried that I might develop benzodiazepine dependence. This GP decided to write a management plan for hypertension and prescribed an antihypertensive drug. I told him I did not want to take it because I did not believe that I had developed hypertension, since I led a healthy lifestyle and did not have other predisposing factors. He said that antihypertensive drugs could reduce my blood pressure and slow down my heart rate and that, unlike benzodiazepines, they are not addictive. I decided not to take the prescribed medication. I have since learned that heart palpitations are a common sign of perimenopause that are "probably not an indication of heart disease" and do "not usually lead to serious problems" (Zala, Swan, and Prior 57). Had either of my doctors explained this to me, I would not have gone to such extreme lengths to determine a diagnosis and find a cure.

But at the time, I did not know about palpitations being a normal perimenopausal symptom, and I worried about my health and my life. I became isolated and engulfed in depressive thoughts about what would happen next. My father's death and my husband's frequent surgeries contributed to my worries. Grief related to my father's death was not completely resolved. He died just a few days before his ninety-third birthday. As a Christian, I knew he was now with God, but I missed him. At some point, most everyone experiences the futility of life, but my sense of nearness to death might have contributed to my worries. I viewed my bodily changes as indicative of the end of life rather than signs of ageing. I wondered whether they would ever end and if I would ever become better. Dillaway writes that uncertainty is a common feeling experienced by women in this stage ("When Does Menopause Occur" 37), but it was overwhelming in my case. This was the stage of arguing with God: Why? Why is this happening to me? What have I done wrong? I was jealous of other people's good health. I felt sad looking out the window to see older neighbour ladies walking with their dogs in the morning and evening. I wondered: "Will my palpitations cease? Will I be able to walk around the street as these elderly ladies do?" I questioned the meaning of life, perceived my ill health as underserved punishment, and felt that God had abandoned me. Experiencing a heightened sense of the inevitability of death, I invested in prayers and asked God's forgiveness for the sins of my life.

I was unhappy that Australian doctors were unable to provide a definitive diagnosis of my health issues, particularly concerning the palpitations, tachycardia, and the unexplainable rise of my blood pressure. They failed to link these symptoms with perimenopause. I was lost; sinus tachycardia was not an answer to me. As a health professional, I wanted to know the cause of my symptoms. If there was nothing wrong with my heart, then why did I have palpitations and tachycardia and why did I need to undertake repeated tests? As a clinician, I thought that having a clearer diagnosis would have been more helpful, although I realize that the menopausal transition is not an illness. I lost my trust in conventional medicine and clinicians and relied on self-diagnostics. Again, I did not link these symptoms with perimenopause but with something serious. I initially thought the palpitations were a side effect of Diclofenac—a nonsteroidal anti-inflammatory drug prescribed to me to manage pleurisy—or they were related to postviral infection vasomotor reactions, to age-related cardiovascular changes, or to a generalized anxiety disorder related to my family circumstances. I found it so difficult to see that some of my bodily changes, such as fatigue, were related to perimenopause. I linked it with my extensive parenting and caregiving commitments. I attributed hot flushes, night sweats, and severe chills to my frequent episodes of flu. Compared with the palpitations, tachycardia, and increased blood pressure, these symptoms were a nuisance rather than a worry.

After a few months, I noticed the pattern: Palpitations and other signs occurred or increased a few days before and during the first few days of my period. This was my first realization that these changes could be hormone related. I tried to talk to my mum, but she had not had any of the perimenopausal changes I was experiencing. She said there is no such thing as menopausal transition—you just stop having your periods. I asked my GP if my symptoms could be related to perimenopause and if I could check my follicle-stimulating hormone (FSH) and luteinizing hormone (LH), which were tests my medical training had taught me were useful for assessing hormonal levels in perimenopause. He told me these tests were no longer used because they were no longer considered to be indicative of menopause, given that the levels of hormones fluctuate on a daily basis.

In frustration, I started to read the biomedical literature, which focused on explanations of hormonal changes in the perimenopausal period and related signs and symptoms. I was relieved to make connections between my symptoms and the perimenopausal symptoms discussed in the literature. However, I looked for but did not find information about whether or not my symptoms would cease once I reached menopause. I wanted to know if they would all go away and when. I also wanted to know how to reduce their frequency and severity. All the health-promoting suggestions—reduce alcohol intake, stop smoking, avoid coffee and sugary drinks, eat healthy food, lose weight, and talk to your doctor—I followed already. I was annoyed with these repetitive suggestions, although I realized they could be helpful to women who did not follow these recommendations. I turned to online women's forums for answers and came to value women's experiences of perimenopause. First, I wanted to find out if other women experienced the same issues and what they did to manage them (Ziebland and Wyke 230). Second, I wanted to know if there were any reports that these symptoms reduced once menopause arrived. I found out that other women with palpitations and tachycardia made needless trips to the emergency department. There was a lot of uncertainty in women's accounts and a heightened sense of dissatisfaction with health services.

My former supervisors, my current senior colleagues, anthropologists, and women's health researchers, were first to associate my palpitations with possible perimenopausal changes. Their explanations helped me to arrange the interlocking puzzle pieces of my symptoms and feelings into a complete picture of perimenopause. I am grateful for their private messages to me and suggestions to rest. I am also grateful to church elders who visited me, prayed with me, and prayed for me.

I am thankful to my husband, who not only is a medical doctor, family planning specialist, public health professional, and medical educator but also a loving and caring man. My husband went through perimenopause by my side. One day, he said: "I know that you would not listen to me; but I want you to drink this. My mum used to drink this all the time; all women in Eritrea drink this." The warm drink he prepared for me was made of toasted and ground linseed. Whether it was the plant-based estrogens in the mixture, the placebo effect, or a combination of both, I became better on the same day. My heart rhythm slowed down and my palpitations reduced. I remember calling him to ask: "Can you please bring me another bottle of the linseed drink when you come to pick me up from work?"

Late Perimenopause

I describe this late perimenopausal stage I am in now, in my early fifties, as one of stability: employment stability, financial stability, family stability, stability in relationships, and, most importantly, perimenopausal stability. My blood flow has significantly reduced, and the time between bleeding episodes has increased. Every time my period is a few days late, I think, "Oh, it is probably the beginning of menopause," but it is not. I occasionally have palpitations at the beginning of my period or when I feel stressed. When I do, I describe them as mild, short, and nonfrightening. I have become less worried about them. I still have a few hot flushes in the morning and, occasionally, when I am cooking or if I sit in front of a heater. I have mild urine leakage prior to my periods, but this is easily managed with light bladder leakage pads. I have not yet experienced vaginal dryness; possibly, it will come when I reach menopause. I have no changes in sexual function. The frequency of sex may have reduced compared to the time my husband and I first met, but it has definitely increased compared to the midstage of perimenopause. The assurance and joy I find in my family and work commitments, good health, time for hobbies, and improved general wellbeing contribute to my sexual function and satisfaction.

My desire to be attractive has returned. I eat well, dress well, and use cosmetic products. I feel healthy, and I work hard. I enjoy everything that I do, including taking care of my garden and other activities I loved doing in the early stage of my perimenopausal transition. I love my grandchildren, and they love me. Our eldest daughter and her husband have blessed us with three granddaughters, ages ten, nine, and two. They live in Tasmania but spend most of their school holidays with us. Those days are filled with trips to markets, second-hand shops, playgrounds, and parks. We have time for gardening, dancing, and outdoor family competitions—all fun activities that we feel we missed doing with our children as frequently as we should have. I see my delightful ten-month-old grandson at least twice a week. My middle daughter and son-in-law lived with us until recently when they moved into their own home a twenty-minute drive away. I miss the daily contact with my grandson but have come to appreciate their visits even more; I am always eager to feel his tiny hands around my neck. I enjoy the present, and I do not worry about the future.

Conclusions

All women who naturally transition to menopause will go through stages of perimenopause. For some, it may seem like three stages; for others, it may seem like five or seven. As with preadolescence, or any other life stage, not all women will experience perimenopause in the same way. In this chapter, I have discussed my own staged experience of perimenopause and have described in detail the social, cultural, psychological, and religious factors that have shaped my experience. I have also provided a detailed description of changes in my body, mind, and spirit during early-, mid-, and late-stage perimenopause. Considering both nonphysical and physical factors, I believe, enriches the holistic understanding of this transition. I suggest that a complex theory of menopausal transition—one that brings together biomedical and holistic perspectives—should be developed so that both women and clinicians can better recognize and understand the mind, body, and spirit elements of the transition.

These various perspectives are reflected in a variety of existing definitions of menopausal transition. For example, Marianne Ammitzboll reflects upon the biological perspective and describes the menopausal transition as "a natural rite of passage" (107) related to the biological "phases according to whether we bleed or not: from birth to menarche; from menarche to menopause; and from menopause to death" (56). Justine Coupland and Angie Williams discuss the sociopolitical and gender perspective and describe it as a passage to freedom and emancipation (419), and Bobbie Crumbley highlights the religious perspective and refers to the menopausal transition as "a God given rite of passage" (1). She believes that God shapes women's experiences of this period and "uses medicine, hospitals, and various treatment modalities to bring about healing" (3). Her description reflects my personal current view of this transition.

My other suggestion is to avoid dichotomizing perimenopausal attitudes and experiences as either positive or negative. Taking into account all aspects of women's lives— including the various social, cultural, psychological, and hormonal factors that may shape them—and given that this transition occurs over a lengthy period of time, women can expect to experience both positive and negative changes in different stages of perimenopause. Even the same symptom can be perceived by women differently. One woman may experience hot flushes as positive because she is always cold, whereas another may perceive them as annoying or sleep disturbing. Rereading my own work, I still do not know if my discussion of sub stages would be different if my father had died earlier or later than he did or if I had not miscarried and had a much-wanted child.

Such uncontrollable variables contribute to each woman's unique experience of perimenopause. Our experiences can be described as changes, signs, or symptoms. My health issues related to hormonal changes in midstage are best understood as symptoms. However, these symptoms were not linked with perimenopause by either myself or the health professionals involved in my care. Uncertainty related to underdiagnosis and unpredictability of health outcomes affected my mood and limited my ability to decide on how to manage these perimenopausal symptoms as I was experiencing them. I hope that some women will find my detailed explanation helpful in reducing their own fears and concerns related to the perimenopausal transition.

Finally, I do not want to blame health professionals for how little they helped me through this transition. Women's experiences of peri-menopause are "heterogeneous" and "fluid," which are related to factors shaping these experiences (Chirawatkul and Manderson 1545). Multiple signs and symptoms of the perimenopausal transition, and the severity of these signs and symptoms, as well as women's varying explanations of their experiences, may impede health professionals' understanding of this transition.

I am a health professional, yet I misinterpreted perimenopausal symptoms that I experienced, attributing them to an unknown serious illness. I would not have worried about my health if my symptoms were minimal or typical of how many others experience perimenopause, with hot flushes, night sweats, and missed periods. I was never asked about, nor did I discuss with the doctors, I saw my difficult social circumstances, including my recent miscarriage, my father's death, my husband's surgeries, and my related grief and fear of what would happen next. Being most concerned about my cardiovascular symptoms, I did not talk to them about the changes I noticed in my mental and reproductive health. They were not aware of my psychological state and spiritual concerns, nor did they have complete information about my physical health, including my menstrual problems. We all missed the bigger picture. I believe greater awareness—by both women and their clinicians—of the mind, body, and spirit elements related to this life stage is vital for early recognition and effective support for the perimenopausal transition.

Works Cited

Ammitzboll, Marianne. *Menopause: A Natural Rite of Passage. Women's Voices at Midlife*. Institute of Transpersonal Psychology, 1991.

Chirawatkul, Siriporn, and Lenore Manderson. "Perceptions of Menopause in Northeast Thailand: Contested Meaning and Practice." *Social Science & Medicine*, vol. 39, no. 11, 1994, pp. 1545-54.

Coulter, Angela. "Understanding the Experience of Illness and Treatment." *Understanding and Using Health Experiences: Improving Patient Care*, edited by Sue Ziebland. Oxford, 2013, pp. 7-15.

Coupland, Justine, and Angie Williams. "Conflicting Discourses, Shifting Ideologies: Pharmaceutical, 'Alternative' and Feminist Emancipatory Texts on the Menopause." *Discourse & Society*, vol. 13, no. 4, 2002, pp. 419-45.

Crumbley, Bobbie N. *Pause and Celebrate: Educational Pastoral Approach to Understanding Menopause and Andropause as God Given Rites of Passage*. United Theological Seminary, 2013.

Salis, Isabel de, et al. "Experiencing Menopause in the UK: The Interrelated Narratives of Normality, Distress, and Transformation." *Journal of Women & Aging*, vol. 30, no. 6, 2017, pp. 520-40.

Dillaway, Heather. "Menopause Is the 'Good Old': Women's Thoughts About Reproductive Aging." *Gender & Society*, vol. 19, no. 3, 2005, pp. 398-417.

Dillaway, Heather. "When Does Menopause Occur, and How Long Does It Last? Wrestling with Age and Time-Based Conceptualizations of Reproductive Aging." *NWSA Journal*, vol. 18, no. 1, 2006, pp. 31-60.

Fairhurst, Eileen. "'Growing Old Gracefully' as Opposed to 'Mutton Dressed as Lamb': The Social Construction of Recognising Older Women." *The Body in Everyday Life*, edited by Sarah Nettleton and Jonathan Watson. Routledge, 1998, pp. 258-75.

Gold, Ellen B. "The Timing of the Age at Which Natural Menopause Occurs." *Obstetrics and Gynecology Clinics of North America*, vol. 38, no. 3, 2011, pp. 425-40.

Gordon, Jennifer L., et al. "Naturally Occurring Changes in Estradiol Concentrations in the Menopause Transition Predict Morning Cortisol and Negative Mood in Perimenopausal Depression." *Clinical Psychological Science: a Journal of the Association for Psychological Science*, vol. 4, no. 5, 2016, pp. 919-35.

Gordon, Judith R., Joy E. Beatty, and Karen S. Whelan-Berry. "The Midlife Transition of Professional Women with Children." *Women in Management Review*, vol. 17, no. 7, 2002, pp. 328-41.

Harris, Margaret. "Aging Women's Journey toward Wholeness: New Visions and Directions." *Health Care for Women International*, vol. 29, no. 10, 2008, pp. 962-79.

Hunter, Myra, and Melanie Rendall. "Bio-Psycho-Socio-Cultural Perspectives on Menopause." *Best Practice & Research Clinical Obstetrics & Gynaecology*, vol. 21, no. 2, 2007, pp. 261-74.

Lock, Margaret, and Patricia Kaufert. "Menopause, local biologies, and cultures of aging." *American Journal of Human Biology*, vol. 13, 2001, pp. 494-504.

O'Reilly, Andrea. "Introduction." *Feminist Mothering*, edited by Andrea O'Reilly. State University of New York Press, 2008, pp. 1-22.

Prior, Jerilynn C. "Clearing Confusion About Perimenopause." *BC Medical Journal*, vol. 47, no. 10, 2005, pp. 534-38.

Samouei, Rahele, and Mahboubeh Valiani. "Psychological Experiences of Women Regarding Menopause." *International Journal of Educational and Psychological Researches*, vol. 3, no. 1, 2017, pp. e1-e5.

Team, Victoria. "Midlife Burnout: Mothering, Multiple Roles, and Multiple Losses." *Middle Grounds: Essays on Midlife Mothering*. Eds. Kathy Mantas, and Lorinda Peterson, Demeter Press, 2018, pp. 147-64.

Ziebland, Sue, et al. "Examining the Role of Patients' Experiences as a Resource for Choice and Decision-Making in Health Care: A Creative, Interdisciplinary Mixed-Method Study in Digital Health." *Programme Grants for Applied Research*, vol. 4, no. 17, 2016, pp. 1-214.

Ziebland, Sue, and Sally Wyke. "Health and Illness in a Connected World: How Might Sharing Experiences on the Internet Affect People's Health?" *Milbank Quarterly*, vol. 90, no. 2, 2012, pp. 219-49.

Zala, Lissa, Andrea Swan, and Jerilynn C. Prior. *Transitions through the Perimenopausal Years: Demystifying Your Journey*. Trafford Publishing, 2004.

Chapter 17

From the Crowning to the Crone: Extrapolating Judy Chicago's *Birth Project* to Older Women

Anne Barrett

The devaluation of older women and the silence around reproductive aging are reflected in cultural products, including art. Younger female bodies—those of childbearing years and meeting the culture's youthful beauty standards—are more prevalent than older female bodies, even within feminist art. Although aging women's experiences are less visible than younger women's, insight can be gained by viewing feminist art through an aging lens. Taking this approach, I examine one of the most well-known feminist works of art: The *Birth Project* (1980–1985) by Judy Chicago. Involving over 150 women needleworkers and touring over one hundred venues, the artwork in this collection made a revolutionary statement about women's birth experience. It put women's creative power at the centre and highlighted their varied and complex experiences from their own perspectives rather than those of others, including the child and the medical profession.

This chapter examines the broader implications of the *Birth Project* for revisioning women's lives beyond their youth and outside of their reproductive lifecycles. To develop this argument, I draw on two archetypes of women's lives: the mother and the crone. Whereas the *Birth Project* centres on the mother, I extrapolate its messages about women to the crone by exploring parallels between them. With these parallels as a backdrop, I make several observations about Chicago's revisioning of women and provide illustrations of how they could be extended to the crone.

The *Birth Project's* Origin and Expansive Implications

Judy Chicago, one of the leading contemporary feminist artists, created the *Birth Project* in response to her observation of the lack of images of the birth process, particularly those reflecting women's perspectives. As she noted in *Beyond the Flower: The Autobiography of a Feminist Artist*: "When I scrutinized the art-historical record, I was shocked to discover that there were almost no images of birth in Western art, at least not from a female point of view. I certainly understood what this iconographic void signified: that the birth experience (with the exception of the birth of the male Christ) was not considered important subject matter, even to women" (89).

The absence of images led Chicago to create her own "original, woman-centered iconography about the experience," requiring her "to basically start from scratch to invent forms and symbols that could represent what was so obviously a primal human experience" (92). To prepare for the project, Chicago spoke with many women about their birth experiences, surveyed more than a hundred women, and observed childbirth. She used these materials to create images that dozens of women across the United States, Canada, and New Zealand stitched, using multiple techniques, including embroidery, batik, crochet, and quilting. The result was a collection of drawings, prints, paintings, and needlework pieces celebrating "the birth-giving capacity of women along with their creative spirit" ("Birth Project (1980–1985").

Although the *Birth Project* centres on a particular event within many women's early adulthood, its revisioning of women has implications extending far beyond this stage of their reproductive lives. I see this expansiveness symbolized in the images themselves—for example, in the energetic, undulating, and outwards-reaching lines in the collection's signature piece, *The Crowning* (Figure 1). Chicago's writings about the *Birth Project* allude to this more expansive meaning. For example, in her book *The Birth Project*, chronicling the project's genesis and course, she writes: "As I listened and studied and read, I realized that it was not only birth I was learning about, but also the very nature of these women's lives, and that both of these subjects were shrouded in myth, mystery, and stereotype. I knew that I wanted to dispel at least some of this secrecy" (6).

In journals kept during the project, the needleworkers also alluded to the project's far-reaching effects, particularly in their own lives. Stitcher Gwen Glesmann says the following:

> I had trouble relating to my [assigned] image for a long time. Not having any children or any plans for having children, the image did not inspire any special feelings in me. However, my whole involvement in stitching this piece became a celebration of my own rebirth and the incredible joy of bringing myself out of the oppressive roles I have been taught. (*The Birth Project* 36)

Similarly, stitcher Candis Duncan Pomykala says: "The piece I worked on came to be synonymous with my personal growth and a formal statement of my refusal to accept the expectations imposed on me" (149). Another stitcher, Maria Lo Biondo, references the project's potential to spark broader social change: "It seems that being part of the *Birth Project* has unleashed our energies in many ways. Who would have dreamed that a 'sewing circle' would become so revolutionary!" (148).

The project's expansion beyond the birth experience also has a temporal quality, as its themes have applicability across historical and personal dimensions of time. I see its link with historical time reflected in the *Creation of the World* (Figure 2). The works in this series reflect Chicago's desire to move beyond the patriarchal creation myths of Western culture, particularly the Judeo-Christian depiction of men creating life. She wanted "to make the creation of the universe an intimately feminine act" (*The Birth Project* 13). She succeeds, as needle-worker Gerry Melot describes: "The image is of a woman lying on her back giving birth to the world; it is a very powerful image of womanhood, an image that is not seen very often. It tells a new story of creation while still incorporating the theory of evolution; there is a sea with fish that become the sky and birds which in turn become the infinity of space" (18). The images also allude to temporal expansiveness within women's lives. For example, *Birth Trinity* (Figure 3) depicts three figures, inter-connected in a way suggestive of either cross-generation linkages or women's development across their life stages. Further references to women's life stages, particularly those beyond the reproductive years, are found in Chicago's descriptions of the needleworkers: "The age range of the group was striking; there were young women who had benefited from the changes in attitude that had produced the alternative birth movement, and there were also women the age of their mothers and, in some cases, their actual mothers" (24).

The *Birth Project*'s applicability across women's lives also is referenced in Chicago's description of "birth and its subsequent responsibilities [as] metaphor for being 'caught' by the life process, something most women seem to both crave and fear" (*The Birth Project* 34). I suggest that this theme has relevance across women's lives, as they are "caught" in not only a reproductive lifecycle but also a broader lifecycle, which for most women spans decades beyond their fertile years. Indeed, women's longevity advantage drives much of population aging, with women constituting 70 per cent of Americans ninety or older (Ortman et al. 25). However, they spend a higher proportion of their lives with physical impairments than men do (Solé-Auró et al. 10). These patterns, in conjunction with women's greater responsibility for caring for both younger and older family members, resonate with Chicago's observations about women's life process and their reflection in the *Birth Project*.

Archetypes of Women's Lives: Parallels Between Mother and Crone

The *Birth Project*'s applicability to women's lives beyond their repro-ductive years can be further illuminated by an analysis of the three archetypes of women's lives drawn from matriarchal belief systems: the maiden (symbolizing creation), the mother (preservation), and the crone (destruction). In particular, although the *Birth Project* deals with the mother archetype, I extrapolate its messages about women to the crone.

Both mother and crone were central archetypes in our prepatriarchal past. The mother was accorded status as the giver of life. The crone, too, had a valued status in many cultures of antiquity. Rather than the current dominant associations that are purely negative, the crone had positive associations in matriarchal belief systems. Writing about the crone in antiquity, Barbara Walker describes her as a "healer, judge, wisewoman, arbiter of ethical and moral law, owner of sacred lore, mediator between the realms of flesh and spirit and—most of all the functions of the Crone—the funerary priestess and Death Mother, controlling the circumstances of death as she controlled those of birth" (32). She was viewed as drawing her wisdom and strength from her menopausal status—namely, her retained menstrual blood, a theory found in seventeenth-century discussions of witchcraft (Gifford 26).

These archetypes were also interconnected, with the crone viewed as an integration and culmination of the cycle of creation, preservation, and destruction. Goddess mythology often reflected this interconnection. For example, the Mycenaean Demeter was "a trinity collectively named Mother De, that is, the delta or triangle, a basic female symbol throughout the ancient world" (Walker 24). Moreover, each point of Demeter's triangle was originally personified: "There was Kore the Virgin, Pluto the Mother, and Persephone the Crone" (Walker 24). Reflecting a view of "existence as *becoming*, not *being*," (Walker 33), the mother and crone are linked in a cycle of continual development produced by (and producing) an interplay between their light and dark sides. As Ruth Ray describes, the light side of the mother archetype encompasses "nourishment, creativity, generativity, and illumination through relationships," whereas the dark side reflects "manipulation and the use of relational power to abandon, control, and destroy others" (111). Turning to the crone, her light side contains "self-knowledge and self-mastery, assertiveness, strength, courage, integrity, and wisdom"— which is countered by her dark side of "impatience with those who are less insightful and the use of spiritual powers to control and manipulate" (111).

Patriarchal culture, however, obscures the idea of interconnectedness over the lifecycle and the notion of continual lifelong growth. As Walker writes: "Instead of aging normally through their full life cycle, women are constrained to create an illusion that their growth process stops in the first decade or two of adulthood" (31). The *Birth Project*, too, focuses on this short life stage and rarely includes images of older women as midwives, although an exception is found in *Mother India*, which depicts a birth attended by two older women. Midwifery was a traditional role for the crone and one that links women across generations—a linkage that is illustrated, for example, by the "granny midwives" of the southern states who attended most African American births in the late 1800s through to the mid-1900s (Varney and Thompson 10). Although younger women are the focus of *Birth Project* images, the needleworkers themselves represent a much wider age range, and the stitchers' comments reflect a linking of mother and crone. An example is provided by stitcher Mary Kidd Fogel's journal entry: "My feelings about our woman/quilt are strong earth feelings. They tangle endlessly with my grandmother's spirit and life, as well as with my own relationship with her" (*The Birth Project* 82).

These archetypes also share a radical alteration, even burial, by patriarchal institutions. Patriarchal religion erased goddesses and marginalized the mother figure, replacing her with a heavenly father. Discussing her research on creation myths across time and around the world, Chicago observes the "gradual changeover from matriarchal societies (reflected in myths featuring the female as a source of life) to patriarchal civilizations like the Judeo-Christian one we've inherited (mirrored in myths about 'God the Father' creating 'Man')" (*The Birth Project* 11). Patriarchy also negated women's role in the birth process through a medicalization process, which shifted power from midwives, often older women, to mostly male doctors (Wertz and Wertz 46). The crone was eradicated through the usurping of older women's authority, and "crone" became a derogatory term. In his historical analysis of terminology for older adults, Herbert Covey reveals that references to "hag" with negative connotations date back to the 1300s. Noting that the use of crone is similar to that of hag, he observes that "this tone has carried over to the way older women have been perceived and treated in succeeding eras" (295). As Walker explains, "The gray-haired high priestesses, once respected tribal matriarchs of pre-Christian Europe, were transformed by the newly dominant patriarchy into minions of the devil" (30). Reflecting this shift, the history of midwifery in the United States reveals that witch hunting in New England often centred on midwives, particularly those who had attended the birth of a stillborn or deformed infant (Varney and Thompson 9).

These archetypes were also rediscovered by second-wave feminists, like Chicago. Regarding birth, second wavers advocated a reorientation that emphasizes women's control over their own experiences (Brubaker and Dillaway 35). Crone, too, was rediscovered and can be seen in the emergence of a women's spirituality movement, aimed at retrieving prepatriarchal goddess worship and reintroducing the crone to Western culture (Manning 102). Yet this change has been less widespread. We have so far seen more woman-centred birth experiences than croning ceremonies. With these parallels between mother and crone as a backdrop, I make three broad observations about Chicago's revisioning of women and illustrate how they could be extended to the crone.

Birthing and Aging Bodies Made Visible

The *Birth Project*'s defining characteristic is that it makes women's creative power visible, thus confronting the viewer with its reality. As stitcher Gerry Melot explains: "There is a feeling of power and strength about each piece. It says: This is woman in her natural state, using her tremendous capability for creation" (*The Birth Project* 83). The collection also makes visible the broader contexts within which individual women's birth experiences are located. Chicago foreshadows this consequence of her work when she writes: "It seemed to me that another consequence of the absence of images was that women are not provided a way of seeing the birth experience in its larger, more universal dimension. It was striking that no woman I interviewed ever discussed her birth experience from anything but a personal perspective" (*Beyond the Flower* 93). By making visible women's birth experiences, the project resists the culture's view of women's entire reproductive lives, from menarche to menopause, as part of women's unbounded bodies, which should be hidden from view and rarely discussed.

We can contrast the visibility of women in the *Birth Project* with women's invisibility as they age beyond their reproductive years. As Walker writes: "The law doesn't murder witches any longer, but modern society does eliminate older women in a sense. They are made invisible. They rarely appear on those mythic mirrors of our culture, movie and television screens.... In real life also signs of older womanhood are not supposed to be seen" (30-31). These observations are consistent with research documenting the underrepresentation and stereotypical portrayal of older women in film (Lauzen and Dozier; Robinson et al.) and aging women's feelings of invisibility (Barrett et al.; Hurd Clarke).

Women's invisibility is especially striking in deep old age, the stage proximate to death. This most female-dominated of all life stages is spent by many women away from view—isolated at home or in nursing homes. Older women are more likely than older men to report feeling lonely

(Aartsen and Jylhä), and they are more likely to be admitted to a nursing home and spend a longer time there (Martikainen et al.). Their invisibility is also reflected in researchers' more limited interest in this life stage, particularly from the perspective of older adults themselves, as opposed to their care workers. An explanation is suggested by Walker's discussion of patriarchy's erasure of the crone, whose "death-dealing aspect" challenged male authority to grant or deny life, even eternal life (33). The oldest crones "represented the kind of death that our culture wished to conceal, making it invisible as old women are made invisible: the common garden-variety kind of death; death in old age, death from wasting disease, death after slow degeneration of body and mind" (33).

Chicago makes women's experiences visible through not only the *Birth Project* images but also her choice of medium—needlework—which was traditionally viewed as a craft not as art because it was done by women. As Chicago explains, "Needlework was not considered art in any of the art schools I attended ... working in fibers virtually guaranteed that you would not be considered a 'serious artist'" (*The Birth Project* 4). I argue that needlework is further devalued by its greater association with old women, who are often stereotypically depicted knitting in a rocking chair. Chicago elevates this creative activity by insisting it be considered art. Needlework also has been, for most of history and across girls' and women's lives, an activity that was stitched into their daily lives and was fitted around their other responsibilities, as it was for the many needleworkers involved in the *Birth Project*. The competing demands on women's time were reflected in some of the *Birth Project* pieces through the needles left in the work of stitchers withdrawing from the project due to family demands. As Chicago explains: "I decided to present this unfinished work as a symbol for women's uncompleted lives. This image celebrates women's fecundity and her power to bring forth new life. How ironic that this very power often causes us to lose control of our own lives" (63).

Birthing and Aging Bodies Taking up Space

Not only are women's birthing bodies visible in the *Birth Project*, but they also dominate the pieces, challenging the cultural message that women should take up little physical, social, and political space—and even less as they age. These are images of powerful, strong women, as illustrated by *Birth Power* (Figure 4), described by needleworker Sandie Abel as follows: "The aura surrounding the figure seems to radiate the pain away from it, transforming the heat from pain into power" (*The Birth Project* 59). Other needleworkers made similar observations about their pieces, like Dianne Barber who writes: "The first image I worked on was *The Crowning*, and I grew to love it. I was especially fond of the curve of the arms and the way the knees seemed to express the strength required to give birth" (35). Reflecting on the broader message of her image, stitcher Kate CloudSparks writes the following: "Although I have never had a baby, the image has meant my Self to me—she is my universal experience as a woman, and she reassures me by her bigness, her strength, the set of her jaw" (86). The images stand in stark contrast to the lifelong pressure women feel to maintain, or strive towards, thinness—an expectation reflecting the broader mandate to diminish themselves and yield their space to others.

Reflecting the *Birth Project*'s unwavering focus on the birthing woman, many images do not include a child, and in those that do, the woman remains the focus. The women are not relegated to the background by the perspectives or desires of others or by social constructions of womanhood or motherhood. Drawing this orientation a step beyond birthing experiences, the *Birth Project* images contrast with the currently dominant motherhood ideology, intensive mothering, that places children—to whom good mothers are steadfastly devoted and presumed to derive complete emotional satisfaction (Hays)—at the centre. Women's needs and desires are secondary to their children's. Indeed, some of Chicago's conversations with mothers reflected this ideology. As she recounts: "Many women I had talked to had confessed to a whole range of feelings, but they all said they could only admit to the 'negative' ones years later, as they felt too guilty to say anything except 'everything is wonderful'... and the silence on the subject historically isolates every woman in what must be a prison of unexpressed emotion" (*The Birth Project* 29).

The *Birth Project*'s centring of women's experiences also suggests an alternative framing of older women and their bodies, one that claims the spaces to which they are entitled. Such a revisioning would challenge one of the dominant cultural images of older women—the devoted grandmother. Like her daughter, the so-called good mother, the devoted grandmother is pressured to make her own desires and needs secondary to the younger, and sometimes also older, generations (Harrington Meyer). A *Birth-Project*-inspired revisioning would draw into focus the woman, placing her perspective and experiences at the centre. Such a reframing would also encourage a more honest portrayal of women's aging bodies—with the marvel of change rather than the pursuit of stasis at the centre. It would challenge the expectation that their bodies remain unchanged, lest they become "undesirable" and therefore "invisible" (Dillaway, "[Un]changing" 10). Furthermore, this reframing would reduce the anxiety many women feel about their aging bodies, weight gain among the most salient of concerns (Hurd Clarke). This shift would encourage women to direct their energy away from efforts to shrink their physical space and towards expanding their social and political space while being guided by the "wise anger" (Woodward 56) or "energetic anger" (Furman 168) of the crone.

Accompanying the *Birth Project's* focus on women's bodies is a lack of focus on their faces, which contrasts with our culture's emphasis on girls' and women's faces, especially youthful ones—a central determinant of attractiveness. This focus is seen in the countless beauty products promising to defy age and in the increasing use of surgical and nonsurgical cosmetic procedures. As Laura Hurd Clarke notes, the expanding array of nonsurgical options, such as Botox, has increased the affordability of "having work done" while also magnifying the pressure to do so (99-100). Extrapolating the *Birth Project's* deemphasis of faces to the crone could contribute to the creation of a universal, pan-age sisterhood, unmarked either by dewy youthfulness or tell-tale signs of aging.

Birthing and Aging Bodies' Variation within and across Women

The *Birth Project's* centring of women's perspectives reveals variation across women as well as multidimensional tensions within women. The images contrast with the dominant (and unidimensional) cultural and biomedical portrayals of childbirth emphasizing pain, fear, and unpredictability as well as the medical institution's role in controlling them. The *Birth Project*, instead, conveys a struggle with conflicting and shifting emotional and physical experiences. Are they positive or negative? Wanted or unwanted? Creative or destructive? An illustration of this complexity is provided by a comparison of the celebratory character of *The Crowning* (Figure 1) with the despair conveyed by *Smocked Figure* (Figure 5). The images reflect Chicago's approach toward "the moment of birth ... [as] an existential event ... one in which a female is faced with one of life's great challenges: the bringing into being of another human life with all its attendant agony, triumph, and bliss" (*Beyond the Flower* 91). Further explaining her orientation, she writes: "I have approached the subject of birth with awe, terror, and fascination and have tried to present different aspects of this universal experience—the mythical, the celebratory, and the painful" (*The Birth Project* 6). In its portrayal of these facets, the *Birth Project* alludes to the equally complex array of factors—historical, social, economic, and political—producing variation in pregnancy and birthing experiences across women.

Viewing this observation through an aging lens draws our attention to women's varied and complex experiences of menopause and the several decades that often follow this transition. Feminist researchers have shown that women's views of menopause are much more varied than either the dominant cultural view of "the change" or the medical institution's deficit model of it, which collectively constructs menopause as a negative event that diminishes health, attractiveness, and sexual desire. For example, Heather Dillaway finds that rather than viewing menopause negatively, many women see it as the "good old," something that enhances their freedom—although they were not without concerns about estrogen-linked (and widely-publicized) health risks, such as osteoporosis and heart disease ("Menopause is the 'Good Old'"). Furthermore, her research highlights the importance of placing women's perceptions and experiences of menopause within broader contexts, historical and personal, that give them meaning. Intersecting contexts, and the variation they produce across women, are also the focus of her research with collaborators, which reveals race-ethnic and class differences in the meanings and experiences of menopause (Dillaway et al.). This research not only resonates with the *Birth Project*'s insistence that women's own varied and complex perspectives be reflected in the revisioning of women but also alludes to the void of cultural, including artistic, representations of this kind among and within aging women's experiences.

Conclusion

Applying the *Birth Project*'s framing of birthing women to aging women draws into focus a more honest and nuanced portrayal of women's experiences, centred around their own perspectives on aging's many social, psychological, and biological facets. Such a revisioning of older women would encompass the often overlooked positive aspects of aging, particularly how accumulated experiences broaden perspectives as well as enrich and strengthen a woman's life. Such a framing stands in contrast to the "problem of old women" (Gibson 433)—that is, the frailty, dependence, and loss that our culture tends to attribute to them. The *Birth Project*'s frankness in addressing bodies giving birth has implications for how women should view, treat, and live within their aging bodies. Rather than sequester and shame them, we should seek greater acceptance and, indeed, celebrate them as representations of the awe-inspiring cycle of women's lives.

I conclude with Chicago's own words about her aging experience, having worked on the *Birth Project* in midlife: "I feel that I have accomplished what I set out to do at the beginning... now, with two decades of art-making behind me, I feel in control of my forms and in touch with my power and ready to go forward and produce all the work I can" (15). In a sense, through her work that celebrates and centres women's creative potential, the artist herself becomes a crone.

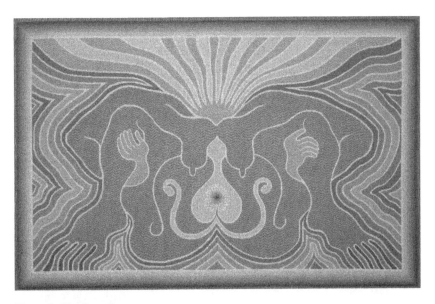

Figure 1: *The Crowning*

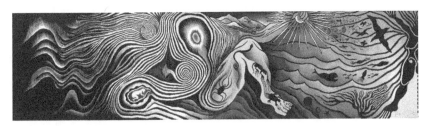

Figure 2: *Creation of the World*

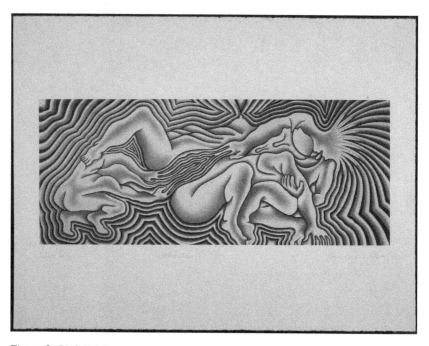

Figure 3: *Birth Trinity*

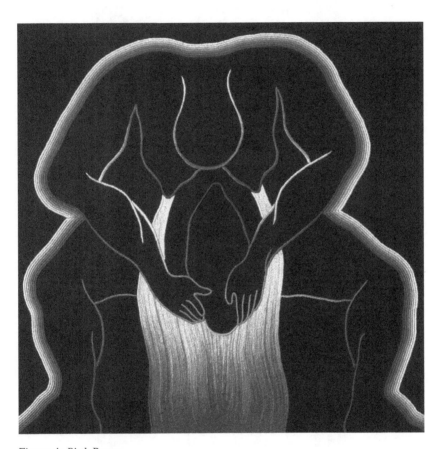

Figure 4: *Birth Power*

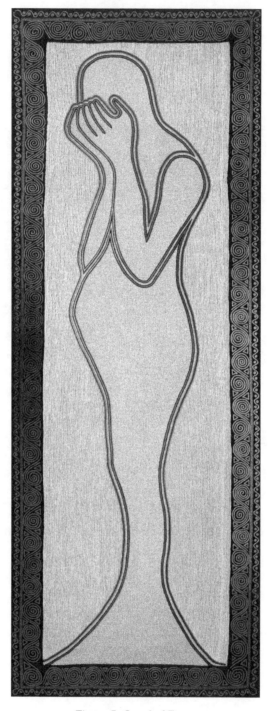

Figure 5: *Smocked Figure*

Works Cited

Aartsen, Marja, and Marja Jylhä. "Onset of Loneliness in Older Adults: Results of a 28-year Prospective Study." *European Journal of Ageing*, vol. 8, no. 1, 2011, pp. 31-38.

Barrett, Anne E., Manacy Pai, and Rebecca Redmond. "'It's Your Badge of Inclusion': The Red Hat Society as a Gendered Subculture of Aging." *Journal of Aging Studies*, vol. 26, no. 4, 2012, pp. 527-38.

Brubaker, Sarah Jane, and Heather E. Dillaway. "Medicalization, Natural Childbirth and Birthing Experiences." *Sociological Compass*, vol. 3, no. 1, 2009, pp. 31-48.

Chicago, Judy. *The Birth Project*. Doubleday & Co., 1985.

Chicago, Judy. *Beyond the Flower: The Autobiography of a Feminist Artist.* New York: Penguin Books, 1996.

Chicago, Judy. "Birth Project (1980–1985)." *Judy Chicago*, www.judychicago.com/gallery/birth-project/bp-artwork/. Accessed 25 Mar. 2018.

Covey, Herbert C. "Historical Terminology Used to Represent Older People." *The Gerontologist*, vol. 28, no. 3, 1988, pp. 291-297.

Dillaway, Heather E. "Menopause is the 'Good Old': Women's Thoughts about Reproductive Aging." *Gender & Society*, vol. 19, no. 3, 2005, pp. 398-417.

Dillaway, Heather E. "(Un)Changing Menopausal Bodies: How Women Think and Act in the Face of a Reproductive Transition and Gendered Beauty Ideals." *Sex Roles*, vol. 53, no. 1-2, 2005, pp. 1-17.

Dillaway, Heather, et al. "Talking 'Among Us': How Women from Different Racial-Ethnic Groups Define and Discuss Menopause." *Health Care for Women International*, vol. 29, no. 7, 2008, pp. 766-81.

Furman, Frida Kerner. *Facing the Mirror: Older Women and Beauty Shop Culture*. Routledge, 1997.

Gibson, Diane. "Broken Down by Age and Gender: 'The Problem of Old Women' Redefined." *Gender & Society*, vol. 10, no. 4, 1996, pp. 433-48.

Gifford, Edward S., Jr. *The Evil Eye: Studies in the Folklore of Vision.* Macmillan, 1958.

Harrington Meyer, Madonna. *Grandmothers at Work: Juggling Families and Jobs*. New York University Press, 2014.

Hays, Sharon. *The Cultural Contradictions of Motherhood*. Yale University Press, 1996.

Hurd Clarke, Laura. *Facing Age: Women Growing Older in Anti-Aging Culture*. Rowman & Littlefield, 2011.

Lauzen, Martha M., and David M. Dozier. "Maintaining the Double Standard: Portrayals of Age and Gender in Popular Films." *Sex Roles*, vol. 52, no. 7-8, 2005, pp. 437-46.

Martikainen, Pekka, et al. "Gender, Living Arrangements, and Social Circumstances as Determinants of Entry into and Exit from Long-Term Institutional Care at Older Ages: A 6-Year Follow-Up Study of Older Finns." *The Gerontologist*, vol. 49, no. 1, 2009, pp. 34-45.

Ortman, Jennifer M., Victoria A. Velkoff, and Howard Hogan. "An Aging Nation: The Older Population in the United States: Population Estimates and Projections. Current Population Reports, P25-1140." *U.S. Census Bureau*, May 2014, www.census.gov/prod/2014pubs/p25-1140.pdf. Accessed 25 Mar. 2018.

Manning, Lydia K. "Experiences from Pagan Women: A Closer Look at Croning Rituals." *Journal of Aging Studies*, vol. 26, no. 1, 2012, pp. 102-08.

Ray, Ruth E. "Toward the Croning of Feminist Gerontology." *Journal of Aging Studies*, vol. 18, no. 1, 2004, pp. 109-21.

Robinson, Tom, et al. "The Portrayal of Older Characters in Disney Animated Films." *Journal of Aging Studies*, vol. 21, no. 3, 2007, pp. 203-13.

Solé-Auró, Aïda, Hiram Beltrán-Sánchez, and Eileen M. Crimmins. "Are Differences in Disability-free Life Expectancy by Gender, Race, and Education Widening at Older Ages?" *Population Research and Policy Review*, vol. 34, no. 1, 2015, pp. 1-18.

Varney, Helen, and Joyce Beebe Thompson. *A History of Midwifery in the United States: The Midwife Said Fear Not*. New York: Springer, 2016.

Walker, Barbara. *The Crone: Woman of Age, Wisdom, and Power*. San Francisco: Harper & Row, 1985.

Wertz, Richard W., and Dorothy C. Wertz. *Lying In: A History of Childbirth in America*. Yale University Press, 1989.

Woodward, Kathleen. "Against Wisdom: The Social Politics of Anger and Aging." *Journal of Aging Studies*, vol. 17, no. 1, 2003, pp. 55-67.

Chapter 18

All New Panties

Cayo Gamber

I always was a big girl, and today I am an old(er) big woman. When I was a big girl, I could fit into the biggest size pair of underwear available at the store: the L underwear. I feared outgrowing L, as there weren't XL sizes widely marketed at that time. I was relieved that I even could fit into my L underwear when I wore a thick menstrual pad attached to an awkward menstrual belt. In fact, if the panties were a bit snug with the thick pad, it was fine because the-almost-too-tight-fit helped to keep the pad in place.

Nonetheless, there always were accidents. I was a sanitary pad girl and then a woman. As a result, I learned to wear black pants. In fact, now, I always wear black pants. Even when choosing my wedding outfit, I said I wanted to wear a tunic and black pants. My friends who were gathered said, "No black pants on your wedding day." My partner and I married, after twenty-five years together, when gay marriage was finally legalized in the United States. Things went awry with my wedding outfit, and in the end, I wore a tunic with black pants. It seemed fitting. I firmly believe when things go awry, whether with menstrual accidents or even wardrobe malfunctions, black pants are always a welcoming and forgiving sartorial choice.

As a middle-aged and then as an old(er) woman, I have worn what my wife and I call "work panties." They are 100 per cent cotton briefs. No hi-cut, no lace, no strings, no thongs, no cut outs. All of my briefs are comfortable and cotton. The reason I wear work panties is due, in large part (excuse the bad pun), to the fact that I went from being a large girl to a fat woman—my size went from L to XL, then XXL, and then to what the fashion industry kindlier calls, albeit sounding a little odd, size twelve. (The size designation is odd because a size-twelve dress and size-twelve underwear are vastly different constructions; one is meant for a woman who weighs 120 pounds, and the other is for a woman who has topped two-hundred pounds.)

For many years, size-twelve underwear were uninspired. They were 100 per cent cotton and came in packets of three colours: white, black, and "nude," which meant a creamy-coffee colour that neither matched the skin tones of white women or women of colour. This was the primary reason we called them work panties; they didn't inspire one to feel playful or sexy. You could choose the white or nude if you were wearing light-coloured clothes and wanted to ensure that the colour of your underwear wouldn't show through. The limited choices meant that you were just wearing very sensible panties that seemed to start just below your breasts and crested at the top of your thighs.

For years, my work panties were stained. It was difficult to invest in new panties when they, too, would just become stained within a month or two. I loved the fact that over time, the pads became thinner and thinner and the adhesive better. I loved the fact that there were long pads that meant you could be protected when sitting down and when standing up. However, even with these changes, there always were stains. They usually occurred overnight.

My mother was someone who would never have tolerated ratty underwear. She would have been embarrassed by mine. If I had to wash my clothes at a public laundromat, I might have taken greater care with my underwear. I also, to be honest, would have taken care to have nicer underwear if the panties that came in my size were fun. Uninspired panties could just become ugly—the elastic could be ratty, and the crotch panel could be stained—but as long as they didn't fall off or ride up in uncomfortable ways, there was no real reason to get rid of such sensible, functional, and not-sexy cotton briefs. So, I just lived with my sensible, less-than-perfect-looking underwear.

I looked forward to menopause because I decided that once menses was safely behind me, I would buy all new underwear and not have to worry about any more stains. Once menopause was assured, I went online and discovered, to my delight, that the choices for women had changed over the years. I spent two hours shopping for underwear. In the end, I still bought 100 per cent cotton briefs, but I was able to find underwear that had fun designs—Mondrian squares, Kandinsky colourful compositions, prosaic plaids, pastels and fluorescents, and even a Hello Kitty, which I loved for the implied double entendre.

I was talking with a small group of friends about menopause, and half of them said they mourned the loss of their menstrual cycles. There would be no more babies in their futures. One or two others, who had decided they did not want to have children, looked forward to menopause. They knew they would no longer need to be concerned about an accidental pregnancy. They also would be free from other people's expectation that they should have children. As one friend said, "I will be able to look at my mother-in-law with feigned sadness and say, 'that time has passed, I am afraid.'" I told them how happy I am to be able to invest in all new panties.

Each morning when I choose a pair of underwear, something that matches my mood or my outfit (not my black pants but the tunics that I favour), I am happy for menopause. I love having panties that stay looking all new for more than one or two months. I love putting on a pair of red and pink polka-dot underwear that make me smile. I think women should celebrate their menopause with a panty party, where they receive all new underwear of their choosing. Each guest should bring the postmenarche honouree one pair to be displayed from an improvised clothesline. Each guest will be asked to add new lines to Jenny Joseph's famous poem that begins:

> When I am an old woman, I shall wear purple
> With a red hat that doesn't go, and doesn't suit me,
> And I shall spend my pension
> on brandy and summer gloves
> And satin sandals,
> and say we've no money for butter....

Their added lines could mention the thrill of new underwear— perhaps purple panties that deserve to be celebrated in purple prose. There will be no airing of dirty laundry; old underwear will be composted discretely after removing the elastic around the waist and legs. And each morning, in the days that follow the panty party, when the postmenopausal woman chooses from her array of new underwear, she will think, "Aren't these briefs with the red and pink roses so delightful and wasn't it lovely of Laura to have chosen them for me." Throughout the day, alone in the bathroom, she will have occasion to look at her rose-patterned panties and to smile with a sense of private joy.

Conclusion

Advancing Our Perspectives on the Menopausal Experience

Heather Dillaway (with Laura Wershler)

The menopausal transition holds both common and unique experiences. Although existing clinical and social science research examines aspects of reproductive aging, researchers often forget to investigate women's everyday, lived experiences of perimenopause and menopause. Women sometimes also forget to unhinge from the "master narratives" (Lyons and Griffin)—the narrow and negative views of the menopausal experience—to think about and engage with this transition for themselves. This volume is an invitation to listen to women as they ponder, ignore, resist, embrace, engage, and experience this life transition, in both real time and on reflection. Our aim as editors was to capture women's diverse musings and adventures, from both personal and scholarly perspectives, with this critical time in the life course. We show both the good and bad feelings, the complete and partial journeys, and the diverse yet also commonplace moments women have across this transition. Our scan of the literature revealed no other recent books that present this multiplicity of women's identities, experiences, and transitions.[1]

The pieces in this volume appropriately showcase women's voices and reflections on the perimenopausal and menopausal transition. As readers move through this collection, they may understandably wonder about the true definition or significance of perimenopause and menopause, since individual authors present, define, and encounter it so differently.

Some authors show us their uncertainties about what perimenopause or menopause is or what it means for them. Others more clearly understand the aspects of their personal identity and experience and the impact of this transition on their own and others' lives. Several authors in this collection show us that the true definition and significance of peri-menopause and menopause can only be understood in retrospect, once women move through and beyond this life stage. We hear from authors about the uncertainties women face while grappling with perimenopause and menopause, and then we catch glimpses of closure and resolution after the fact. In other cases, we do not yet see that closure in authors' reflections. Some authors purposely leave us questioning what menopause is. This is the beauty of a volume like this one. It is a textured collection of snapshots, reflections, and inquiries about living through a reproductive transition—some incomplete and some finished, some out of focus and some sharply defined—representing a broad range of thoughts, identities, and experiences. In this way, these contributions are timeless and when woven together in one volume bring us closer to understanding the intricate and intriguing nature of this life stage.

No matter when they arrive amid women's much larger lives, peri-menopause and menopause are both grounding and destabilizing, dis-orienting and clarifying, positive and negative, typical and atypical, habitable and uninhabitable, as well as knowable and unknowable. Many of our authors clearly highlight this duality of experience. This two-sided experience can be jarring for individual women, as they can feel anchored and unanchored simultaneously while travelling through perimenopause and menopause. This transition may also signify the tangible dichotomies between young and old, mother and nonmother, body and mind, reproductive bodies and post- or nonreproductive bodies, ends and beginnings, past and future. Women may feel in step at times and very much out of step in others. They may feel vulnerable but also strong. They may feel trapped in some spaces or moments and unleashed in others. They may fight against or feel connection to others in their lives during this phase. Feelings about perimenopause and menopause simmer alongside both bodily experiences and other life contexts to inform women's reflections.

Menopause marks a reproductive transition that moves women be-yond the biological capacity to bear children. Because it is a bodily reproductive experience, we could define it as narrowly as much of the existing clinical literature has done. Yet, this book shows the need to look at (1) biological, psychological, and social experiences; (2) the existence of multiple and complicated menopausal meanings and identities; and (3) a variety of other life contexts as women traverse this transition. We must expand our conceptualizations of this transition and zoom out on the lived experience of perimenopause and menopause in order to understand it. Indeed, zooming out facilitates an understanding of the "hidden structures" (Gorelick) that bolster certain perceptions, identities, and experiences and allows us to hear women of various ages as they have engaged this transition. "Hidden structures" of medicalization and gendered beauty norms, for instance, are influential in shaping women's uncertainties about perimenopause and menopause.

The Roots of Uncertainty

Uncertainty is a recurring theme throughout this volume. Authors leave no doubt that the events and processes of perimenopause and menopause induce uncertainty. As Dillaway ("Living in Uncertain Times" 253) discusses elsewhere, this time of life involves: "definitional uncertainties, uncertainties about signs and symptoms, uncertainties about aging, and uncertainties about motherhood and changing relationship statuses" (253). Dillaway continues: "Since the hallmarks of perimenopause and menopause are uncertainty and change ... experiencing menopause and reproductive aging is akin to living in uncertain times, and learning to live in and with this uncertainty is part of the everyday experience of this reproductive and life course transition" (253).

Uncertainties can be unsettling and unpleasant as we live through and with them. Questioning whether one is perimenopausal or menopausal, for instance, is an uncomfortable feeling. Since the purpose of medical appointments is to diagnose and treat symptoms, patient-doctor interactions do not ease women's uncertainties about how to navigate daily experiences or confirm when they might be done with this transition. Indeed, doctors are often as uncertain as women about these things. Existing research suggests that women can stop menstruating between their early forties and late fifties and still be in the normal range (Dillaway, "Living in Uncertain Times" 253-54). Not knowing whether you will be age forty-two or fifty-eight, or somewhere in between, when you meet with your last period can be disconcerting. As we know from pieces in this volume, menopause can occur even earlier, before age forty, or later, in the early sixties. Women can experience close to a year of no menstruation, then flip back to have additional periods before returning to a menopausal trajectory. Waiting for periods in general is hard enough, let alone waiting to see if one has had their final period.

When other bodily signs and symptoms burst in to accompany this waiting game, frustration, annoyance, and uncertainty result. As noted in the introduction, perimenopause is when signs or symptoms—such as irregular or heavy bleeding, hot flashes/flushes, skin changes, changes in libido, insomnia, and others—may begin (see also Dillaway, "Living in Uncertain Times" 254). Whether all these symptoms are actually attributable to perimenopause or some other midlife transition is still up for debate. Regardless, women learn quickly from those around them that these bodily changes are clinically and culturally tagged to perimenopause (Fausto-Sterling).

The focus on bodily signs and symptoms stems from medical bias that contributes to women's uncertainty and negativity about perimenopause. Over time, men's control of the practice of science and their establishment of modern medicine caused women's (healthy, normal, and natural) reproductive processes to be defined as mysterious and "deviant" (Dillaway, "Medicalization Survived" 24). As men's bodies and biological processes were defined as the human standard—what Jacquelyn Zita (193) has deemed the "baseline problem"—women's deviance was confirmed by a process of medicalization (Riessman). Medical vocabulary was developed, treatment plans and protocols were defined, and medical experts in women's health were identified (Riessman 4). In this context, the focus of doctor-patient interactions becomes the diagnosis and treatment of problematic symptoms. Negative feelings (or at least uncertainties) about symptoms become commonplace if the focus is on fixing them. Additionally, if science and medicine define women's reproductive time as her normal time, then post- or nonreproductive time must be seen as abnormal. In this scenario, clinicians may concentrate on the erratic nature of reproductive hormones during perimenopause and prescribe treatment regimens to replace or stabilize those hormones. Exposure to the perspective that reproductive aging is abnormal may contribute to individual women feeling jarred and confused at the onset of this reproductive transition.

The cultural landscape surrounding perimenopause and menopause gets even more complex. Gendered cultural norms about physical appearance may also lead women to feel uncertainty and think negatively about bodily changes. For instance, some signs and symptoms challenge women's ability to control their physical bodies in key moments. Susan Wendell suggests that, as a culture, we believe "it is possible [to] have the bodies we want," and that we should prevent, mask, or postpone bodily change of any kind as much as possible (93–94). Thus, a body that leaks (e.g., sweats or bleeds), changes colour (e.g., becomes flushed), or changes to the touch (e.g., dry or flabby skin) will be seen as "uncontrollable," "disruptive," and "misbehaving" (Dillaway, "Menopausal and Misbehaving" 198). The physical sensation of symptoms like a hot flash/flush or heavy bleeding is only one part of women's symptom experience. They may also worry about how to handle potentially visible symptoms. What should women do if others see their flushed or sweaty skin or notice a menstrual leak? Such happenings can be considered normal within the context of perimenopause, but they also violate gendered cultural norms about beauty and bodily control and signify an aging body (perhaps, even a woman "past her prime," as Mary Jane Lupton notes). A bodily sign or symptom that others can see may feel abnormal, disruptive, and negative. Doctors rushing to treat these observable symptoms also contribute to the uncertainty and negativity women experience. Seeking comprehensive knowledge of women's experiences of symptoms in the everyday and broad understanding of the influences of medicalization and gender norms is crucial if we want to appreciate the reasons for women's uncertainties.

Challenging Existing Perspectives and Moving Beyond Narrowness and Negativity

We must push past the focus on biological or physiological change to think also about the broader psychological and social aspects of this transition. What women live through is not only the physical experience of perimenopause and menopause but a complex reproductive aging transition that can sometimes span decades. Women's identities, perspectives, connections to their bodies, and sense of agency may all change during this transition. Maybe this is its true significance. Confusion and uncertainties, arising from both physical and psychological disruptions, are the means by which women pass through this life-defining stage to arrive at new identities and experiences. Instead of allowing master narratives to define who they are, women can embrace their uncertainties and interpret their transitions more personally. Perhaps this means we need to consider that women's feelings of flux, duality, and uncertainty are not only normal and natural but necessary during this reproductive transition. Maybe this is true throughout their reproductive lives in general.

Recentring, acknowledging, and welcoming the uncertainties at the core of perimenopausal and menopausal experience could be a bold, contemporary approach to helping women thrive during this inevitable transition. A lifetime of reproductive experiences already accustom women to change and uncertainty. During this life transition, as well as before and after, they also have a chance to redefine themselves and their bodies. As Dillaway notes elsewhere: "Thinking about ourselves as living *in* this uncertain time necessarily, rather than just getting *through* it, may be the first step to understanding and owning the impact of menopause and reproductive aging. Individual women, as well as women as a whole, can make what they want of this uncertain time" ("Living in Uncertain Times" 265).

Perhaps not surprisingly, few authors in this volume focus only on symptoms and treatments, suggesting that women are seeking and already using a much broader perspective through which to experience and understand this transition. Several pieces show that both women and doctors may be recognizing the limits to medical knowledge about perimenopause and menopause. For instance, it is now common for health professionals to tell women that menopause is natural and normal, even if they also suggest that menopause causes negative health effects (Meyer). At the very least, there is clinical recognition that a strictly medicalized view of menopause is faulty. This leaves room for feminist refutation of the medicalization of menopause and the impact of gendered beauty norms and brings us towards women's narratives about the broad nature of this life change, even if we know these norms hang like ghosts in the background of women's experience. Our authors push us towards more comprehensive viewpoints and encounters with this transition.

It is interesting to think about whether women must go through uncertainty, and perhaps negativity, to get to the good of menopause. Do the positives in this transition only come from women's willingness to do the hard work of reinventing themselves, finding new purposes, getting through what for some can be physically and psychologically unsettling? Perhaps. At least some authors in this volume show us glimpses of positivity in thinking and in experience. Maybe if women had better information about what to expect, they might embrace the transition with all its chaos as not only an adventure, a slog perhaps, but also an opportunity to evolve, grow, and learn as they travel to a new destination. Or maybe this just puts more expectation on women to "make the best of it," "suck it up," and "get on with life?" Yet several stories in this collection attest that women learn during this life transition that it can be positive to be frustrated, to share with others how hampered they feel, and to release burdens through their thoughts and actions. For example, Marie Maccagno releases her burdens through writing and walking in "Finding Bedrock." Sensing and acknowledging all the uncertainty, negativity, and unknowns, could be an important step towards better understanding the transition to menopause and the development of a post- or nonreproductive identity.

Difference, Uniqueness, Commonality, and Connection

Importantly, authors in this volume also affirm that unique life contexts and connections to others may determine more of women's individual experiences than the biological and/or physiological bases of reproductive aging (Fausto-Sterling). For instance, they may face medical conditions early on that remove their abilities to make choices for themselves. Their choice of intimate partners may also affect decisions about biological parenthood. If they are unhappy in relationships they may put off having children, or they may find themselves with partners who would rather not have biological children. Alternatively, they may choose to be partner-free, and that also shapes their reproductive choices. As women live through their reproductive life courses, they may even have different notions as to what it means to reproduce and/or what a particular process or life stage like perimenopause or menopause means for them. A person's individual circumstances determine what they experience and how they experience it.

Another theme that ties this volume together is women's relationships to others—other perimenopausal or menopausal women, doctors, researchers, coworkers, mothers, children, and partners—and to their past or future selves. Piece after piece makes clear how connections to others influence or help women make sense, or not, of their reproductive experiences, contributing to broad variation in women's relationships to the menopausal transition itself. They are a community of young and old, mothers and nonmothers, and women at the beginning, middle, and end of reproductive lives. They are also in contact with friends, peers, family members, doctors, and others in their communities, and all help shape their reproductive experiences (for good or bad or both). Authors in this volume also make clear that their relationships with literature, art, media, and other cultural influences can affect their conceptualizations of perimenopause and menopause. We must define reproductive experiences as connected and relational as well as unique and common if we are to understand any stage in the reproductive life course.

Finally, reproductive life courses are ongoing, both for individual women and for communities of women. Borrowing from Adrienne Rich's "lesbian continuum" upon which she says all women reside, we propose that we are all also on a reproductive continuum of sorts, both in our own lives as well as in relation to other women. We are products of past reproductive choices and party to future ones. Perimenopausal women who relate to their mother's or daughter's experiences, for instance, place themselves on a continuum of time and connection. Women may also think towards menopause as they wait for their final menstrual period and think back to when they were younger, linking themselves to a pre- and post-, or even nonreproductive time. Women may specifically compare their perimenopausal time to puberty, since both reproductive stages represent change and uncertainty. They may also be prompted to reflect on motherhood choices upon reaching perimenopause. After menopause, women do not exit reproductive experiences for good, however. They still face gendered constructions of themselves and their bodies that are linked to ideas about the biological capacity to reproduce, risks of reproductive cancers, and changing sexual and relationship experiences. Their families may be bearing and raising children, dealing with infertility, and making decisions for elder care. They may still be mothering adult children and finding new intimate partners. Moving beyond the physical capacity to bear children does not diminish involvement in reproductive decisions and actions for themselves, or for family members and friends.

We are all part of the mosaic of reproductive life. We can look backwards and forwards along a continuum to make sense of our and others' past, current, and future life stages. Anne Barrett's analysis of the parallels between the archetypes of the mother and the crone, or birthing bodies and aging bodies, illuminates this reproductive continuum, as do other authors in this volume who think to the past and future when seeking to define current experience. If we pay attention to all the distinct moments, reflections, and inquiries found in this collection, we can see that perimenopause and menopause mean nothing except in relation to what comes before or after. And in examining perimenopause and menopause specifically, we can also see that women's reproductive time (whether acted upon or not) represents just one part of the reproductive life course. By inviting our contributors to explore the menopausal transition in any way they chose, we learned there is much to be said about this transition that goes far beyond bodily experiences and the end of reproductive capacity. Unleashing ourselves from master narratives to think more deeply about the assemblage of identities and experiences we inhabit throughout a life course is key to understanding women's authentic lived experience in all of its complexity.

So where do we go from here? We urge readers, writers, scholars, and researchers to seek out and share more stories about perimenopause and menopause, especially those that push beyond negativity and confusion. In particular, we would love to see stories about what comes after the uncertainty. How do women conceptualize their own transitional experiences once they settle into menopaused lives? Retrospectively, what do women find out about themselves, their bodies, their daily lives, and their relationships with others after living through and beyond uncertainty? What treasures do women find upon reaching cronehood, the "third age" (Radtke, Young, and Van Mens-Verhulst), or their golden years? Contemplating these and other questions raised by the authors in this volume, we wonder what more there is to learn about reproductive life courses— specifically around identity, experience, and transition—from women on the other side of the menopause milestone.

Endnotes

1. *Writing Menopause: An Anthology of Fiction, Poetry and Creative Nonfiction* (2017), edited by Jane Cawthorne and E. D. Morin, contains an impressive breadth of personal reflections but, by intention, no research or clinical perspectives. *The Slow Moon Climbs: The Science, History, and Meaning of Menopause* (2019) by Susan Mattern takes a sweeping, international look at menopause from prehistory to the present. Her thesis is that menopausal symptoms are culturally not biologically determined. In *Flash Count Diary: Menopause and the Vindication of Natural Life* (2020), Darcey Steinke weaves her personal story with historical research and multidisciplinary commentary, but this book is representative of just one person's narrative. By intertwining personal reflections and scholarly perspectives in *Musings on Perimenopause and Menopause,* we intend to show how thinking about these varied cultural and biological perspectives simultaneously can increase our understanding of reproductive aging and the menopausal transition.

Works Cited

Cawthorne, Jane, and Elaine D. Morin. (Eds.). *Writing Menopause: An Anthology of Fiction, Poetry and Creative Nonfiction.* Inanna Publications, 2017.

Dillaway, Heather. "Living in Uncertain Times: Experiences of Menopause and Reproductive Aging." *The Handbook of Critical Menstruation Studies,* edited by Chris Bobel, et al., Palgrave MacMillan, 2020, pp. 253-68.

Dillaway, Heather. "Medicalization Survived the Women's Health Initiative ... But Has Discourse Opened Up?" *Women's Reproductive Health,* vol. 2, no. 1, 2015, pp. 24-28.

Dillaway, Heather. "Menopausal and Misbehaving: When Women 'Flash' in Front of Others." *Embodied Resistance: Breaking the Rules in Public Spaces,* edited by Chris Bobel and Samantha Kwan. Nashville, Vanderbilt University Press, 2011, pp. 197-208.

Fausto-Sterling, Anne. *Myths of Gender* (Rev. Ed.). Basic Books, 1992.

Gorelick, Sherry. "Contradictions in Feminist Methodology." *Gender & Society,* vol. 5, no. 4, 1991, pp. 459-77.

Lyons, Antonia C., and Christine Griffin. "Managing Menopause: A Qualitative Analysis of Self-help Literature for Women at Midlife." *Social Science & Medicine*, vol. 56, no. 8, 2003, pp. 1629-42.

Mattern, Susan. *The Slow Moon Climbs: The Science, History, and Meaning of Menopause*. Princeton University Press, 2019.

Meyer, Vicki F. "Medicalized Menopause, U. S. Style." *Healthcare for Women International*, vol. 24, no. 9, 2003, pp. 822-30.

Radtke, H. Lorraine, Jenna Young, and Jannekke Van Mens-Verhulst. "Aging, Identity, and Women: Constructing the Third Age." *Women & Therapy*, vol. 39, 2016, pp. 86-105.

Rich, Adrienne. "Compulsory Heterosexuality and Lesbian Existence." *The Lesbian and Gay Studies Reader*, edited by Harry Abelove, Michele Aina Barale, and David Halperin. Routledge, 1993, pp. 227-54.

Riessman, Catherine K. "Women and Medicalization: A New Perspective." *Social Policy*, vol. 14, 1983, pp. 3-18.

Steinke, Darcey. *Flash Count Diary: Menopause and the Vindication of Natural Life*. Picador, 2020.

Utz, Rebecca L. "Like Mother, (Not) Like Daughter: The Social Construction of Menopause and Aging." *Journal of Aging Studies*, vol. 25, 2011, pp. 143-54.

Wendell, Susan. *The Rejected Body: Feminist Philosophical Reflections on Disability*. Routledge, 1996.

Zita, Jacquelyn. "The Premenstrual Syndrome: 'Dis-easing' the Female Cycle." *Hypatia*, vol. 3, no. 1, 1988, pp. 77-99.

Notes on Contributors

Gillian Anderson is a professor and chair of the department of sociology at Vancouver Island University. Her research and teaching interests focus on the study of gender and familial relations, and the sociology of home and women's organizing in neoliberal times. Gillian recently coedited *Sociology of Home: Belonging, Community, and Place in the Canadian Context*, published by Canadian Scholars Press International (2016). Her current work is a collaborative project on mothering, mompreneurship, and precarious labour.

Anne Barrett is a professor of sociology and director of the Pepper Institute on Aging and Public Policy at Florida State University. Her research explores two themes: the effects of social relationships on health in middle and later life as well as the social structural patterning and health consequences of subjective aging.

Georgiann Davis is associate professor of sociology at the University of Nevada, Las Vegas. Her work is at the intersection of sociology of diagnosis and feminist theories. In addition to her book *Contesting Intersex: The Dubious Diagnosis*, she has published across outlets ranging from *Gender & Society*, *The Journal of Clinical Endocrinology & Metabolism*, *The American Journal of Bioethics*, *Ms. Magazine*, and *The Advocate*. Georgiann is the former president of the AIS-DSD Support Group (2014–2015), which is one of the largest intersex support groups in the world, and a past board president for interACT: Advocates for Intersex Youth (2017–2020).

Heather Dillaway is a professor of sociology and an associate dean in the College of Liberal Arts and Sciences at Wayne State University in Detroit, Michigan. Her research focuses on women's perimenopause and menopause experiences and has been published in a range of feminist journals, including *Gender & Society; Sex Roles; Journal of Women & Aging; Healthcare for Women International; Women and Health; Women's Studies: An Interdisciplinary Journal;* and *Feminist Formations.* Heather's work on this reproductive transition, as well as her research into the reproductive health experiences of women with physical disabilities, seeks to highlight women's everyday voices and lived experiences.

Christine Eads is a patient advocate living with primary ovarian insufficiency (POI).

Mindy Fried, PhD, MSW, is a sociologist and author of four books, including *Caring for Red: A Daughter's Memoir* (Vanderbilt University Press) and *Taking Time: Parental Leave Policy and Corporate Culture* (Temple University Press). She taught the course Aging in Society at Brandeis University as well as gender, work, and public policy courses at MIT, Tufts University, and Boston University. As principal of Arbor Consulting Partners, Mindy helps organizations build their capacity and strengthen their programs and policies. Having published extensively on work/family issues, she launched a podcast series on caregiving in 2019 called *The Shape of Care.*

Cayo Gamber, an associate professor of writing and women's, gender, and sexuality studies at George Washington University, teaches a writing course titled Legacies of the Holocaust as well as Introduction to Women's, Gender, and Sexuality Studies. She has published widely in the area of Holocaust studies on topics such as the role of museums as pilgrimage sites and the use of archival photographs in creating "illuminated memory." Further publications include essays about the ways cultural artifacts—such as advertisements for menstrual products or the Barbie doll—are implicated in the creation of Western notions of girlhood and womanhood.

Joanne Gilbert, PhD and Charles A. Dana Professor Emerita of Communication and New Media Studies at Alma College in Michigan, is the author of *Performing Marginality: Humor, Gender, and Cultural Critique.* Her work on humour, advocacy, and the discourse of marginalized voices has appeared in *Women's Studies in Communication, Text and Performance Quarterly,* and many other publications.

Catherine M. Gordon is chief of the Division of Adolescent Medicine at Boston Children's Hospital and professor of pediatrics at Harvard Medical School. Her research focuses on factors that affect bone health in adolescents and young adults, particularly as relates to primary ovarian insufficiency (POI).

Alexandra Hawkey has a master's degree in public health and a PhD from the School of Medicine, Western Sydney University (WSU), Australia. Her doctoral research focused on the sexual and reproductive health of culturally and linguistically diverse women. Alexandra is currently an associate research fellow at the Translational Health Research Institute at WSU. Her areas of research are cancer and fertility, women's sexual health, contraception, menstruation and menopause, with a special interest in working alongside women from marginalized communities.

Yolanda Kauffman, LMSW (licensed master social worker), is a puberty educator, contemplative photographer, and late-stage dementia life enrichment coordinator. She creates and facilitates puberty education groups; and is involved in the menstrual activism and education movement. Her menopause journey began at the age of thirty-two, and this experience is key to her involvement in the menstrual advocacy movement.

Koyel Khan received her PhD from the University of Connecticut in 2020 and is currently an assistant professor of sociology at Tennessee Wesleyan University. Her research interests are at the intersection of gender, body, and embodiment.

Donna J. Gelagotis Lee is the author of two award-winning collections: *Intersection on Neptune* (2019), winner of the Prize Americana for Poetry 2018, and *On the Altar of Greece* (2006), winner of the 2005 Gival Press Poetry Award. Her poetry has appeared in publications internationally, including *Atlantis: A Women's Studies Journal, Descant, Feminist Studies, Mothers and Sons: Centring Mother Knowledge* (Demeter Press, 2016), and *Vallum: contemporary poetry.*

Mary Jane Lupton, PhD, is coauthor of *The Curse: A Cultural History of Menstruation* (1976, 1988) and author of *Menstruation and Psychoanalysis* (1993). Professor emeritus from Morgan State University, Maryland, she has published critical studies of Black women writers Maya

Angelou and Lucille Clifton. Mary Jane also has written a book about Blackfeet novelist James Welch.

Marie Maccagno, MA, is a retired psychotherapist and author of the memoir, *The Chocolate Pilgrim: A Journey to Self-Discovery and Transformation on the Camino de Santiago*. After the publication of her book in 2017, she established her company, Adventures in Writing, to help other women find their inner voices. Marie is passionate about supporting aspiring writers to get their words onto the page, meeting in small groups for inspiration and connection.

Beth Osnes, PhD, is an associate professor of theatre at the University of Colorado and cofounder of SPEAK.WORLD, an approach towards vocal empowerment for women for increased self-advocacy and civic participation. Recent books include *Performance for Resilience: Engaging Youth on Energy and Climate through Music, Movement, and Theatre* (2017) and *Theatre for Women's Participation in Sustainable Development* (2013). Beth is featured in the documentary *Mother: Caring for 7 Billion*.

Janette Perz is a professor of health psychology and director of the Translational Health Research Institute at Western Sydney University, Australia. She is a coeditor of the *Routledge International Handbook of Women's Sexual and Reproductive Health* (2020). In collaboration with Jane Ussher, she has undertaken a significant research program in sexual and reproductive health, including the experience of premenstrual syndrome in heterosexual and lesbian relationships and the development and evaluation of a couple-based psychological intervention for PMS.

Magali Roy-Féquière has published her work in *African American Review, Cave Canem: Anthology XIII*, and *Written Here: The Community of Writers Poetry Review 2015*. With a doctorate in Latin American literature from Stanford University, she teaches gender and women's studies at Knox College, Illinois, and is the author of *Women, Creole Identity, and Intellectual Life in Early Twentieth-Century Puerto Rico* (2004). A daughter of multiple diasporas—from Haiti to Puerto Rico to the United States—Magali is at home in three languages. Her ardent desiderata as a practicing Buddhist is to infuse her poems with non-aggressive perception and movement.

Evelina Sterling, director of Research and Strategic Initiatives and associate professor of sociology at Kennesaw State University, Georgia, worked as a public health researcher and medical sociologist focusing on women's health issues for over twenty-five years. She is the author of six consumer health books, including books addressing polycystic ovary syndrome (PCOS) and primary ovarian insufficiency (POI), and is a board member of the Society for Menstrual Cycle Research.

Victoria Team is a senior research fellow in the School of Nursing and Midwifery at Monash University and a health services research fellow at Monash Partners. She trained as a medical doctor in the former Soviet Union, then practiced in Africa for ten years before immigrating to Australia, where she earned a master's and a doctoral degree in public health. Since completing her doctorate at the University of Melbourne in 2007, Victoria has been involved in research in women's health and, currently, in the field of wound management.

Sylvie Teillay-Gambaudo, formerly an assistant professor of philosophy at the University of Durham, United Kingdom, now lives and works in France. Her research in menopause experience is part of a life-long passion for the study of gender, sexualities, and narratives of marginal experience. She is currently writing articles aiming to define a phenomenology of migrancy.

Jane M. Ussher is a professor of women's health psychology in the Translational Health Research Institute at Western Sydney University, Australia. Her research focuses on examining subjectivity in relation to the reproductive body and sexuality and the gendered experience of cancer and cancer care. She is author of over 250 papers and chapters, and eleven books, including *The Madness of Women: Myth and Experience* (Routledge) and *Managing the Monstrous Feminine: Regulating the Reproductive Body* (Routledge). Jane is also editor of the Routledge *Women and Psychology* book series.

Starr Vuchetich is a patient advocate living with primary ovarian insufficiency (POI).

Laura Wershler brings to her writing decades of work and volunteer experience as a sexual and reproductive health advocate, commentator, and educator. Her work has appeared in various newspapers, journals, online media, and the anthology *Without Apology: Writings on Abortion* *in Canada* (2016). Two personal essays will appear in other anthologies published in 2021. One is from her work-in-progress, a memoir about her role as advocate and companion to her mother in deep old age. While earning a certificate in journalism (2011) from Mount Royal University, Laura discovered a love for editing the words of other writers.